Praise for *Still Me*

"Rebecca Chopp, an extraordinary leader in higher education, has written what is perhaps her best book as a gift to all of us. She tells the story of how she faced a devastating diagnosis—Alzheimer's—with courage and creativity. I expected deep sadness. Instead, I found a brilliant, fierce, confrontational strategy to live a life of joy and meaning. Wow!"

—Donna Shalala, former US Secretary of Health and
Human Services and interim president of The New School

"*Still Me* by Rebecca Chopp is an important and elegant contribution to the mystery of Alzheimer's disease and other dementias. Written from the perspective of a highly accomplished university leader who was diagnosed a few years ago, the book is a guide through diagnosis, acceptance, and living with joy. There are lessons to be learned in this book!"

—Dr. Ann-Charlotte Granholm-Bentley, professor
in the Department of Neurosurgery, University
of Colorado Anschutz Medical Campus

"Rebecca Chopp pairs courage and curiosity in a manner that inspires us to push at the boundaries of what is possible in medicine, as well as in our daily lives. Her resolve is unmatched and inspiring."

—Michael Annichine, CEO of Magee-Womens
Research Institute and Foundation

"In her seminal book, *Still Me*, Rebecca Chopp harmonizes and normalizes how to live positively with the dreaded diagnosis of Alzheimer's disease. Without sugarcoating the journey, she shares her determination to live well in the moment, cherish loved ones, and even find new strengths and talents. She guides us on how to spiritually make peace with what life hands us by not fretting the future even if we know intimately what the disease has in store."

—Meryl Comer, cofounder of UsAgainstAlzheimer's and author of *Slow Dancing With A Stranger: Lost and Found in the Age of Alzheimer's*

"Rebecca Chopp takes us with her on a deeply emotional journey, from the despair of an Alzheimer's diagnosis to the rediscovery of life's purpose while living with the disease. A rural Kansan who reached the heights of leadership at three prominent American universities, Chopp has written a soul-touching book that teaches us that we are not defined by disease but by how we find joy in every moment of every day. She makes it clear that it is possible to live with Alzheimer's without losing yourself."

—George Vradenburg, chairman and cofounder of UsAgainstAlzheimer's and cochair of the Davos Alzheimer's Collaborative

"Rebecca Chopp reveals her soul in *Still Me: Accepting Alzheimer's without Losing Yourself.* Diagnosed at the apex of her outstanding career as a scholar and university president, her story is a startling and candid account of the fear and nightmares that followed and her struggle to find joy and inspiration, in part by developing her untapped and unexpected skill in portraiture. This former dean of Yale Divinity School is at her best when describing how Alzheimer's impacts her spiritual journey and how she explores scholarly writings to identify the courage within herself to live well in this new and unexpected chapter in her remarkable life. This book is a gift to the entire Alzheimer's community—a gift of caring, courage, and remarkable insight."

—James Taylor, president of Voices of Alzheimer's

"Rebecca Chopp's powerful account of her personal journey into the reality of Alzheimer's is a bright and shining gift to the world. Her compelling honesty, practical stories, wise advice, and willingness to plumb the spiritual challenges of remaining *Still Me* makes this moving memoir a must-read for many. As a friend and relative of persons with Alzheimer's, her writing not only changed my understanding of her and many others' experiences of Alzheimer's, it deepened my own self-understanding and faith, causing me to reconsider how I think about identity, embodiment, memory, love, health, relationships, and mortality. Rebecca dares to take us where few others have gone, and she has the courage to write honestly about the depths of life as it befalls us all."

—Rev. Serene Jones, MDiv, PhD, president of Union Theological Seminary

"Through this intimate portrayal of her journey after diagnosis, Rebecca Chopp is changing the way we understand Alzheimer's. Contrary to the stigma the disease carries, Rebecca shows us firsthand what it is like to live with Alzheimer's and thrive. This is a must-read, not only for people beginning the Alzheimer's journey, but also for any doctor treating patients with cognitive symptoms. *Still Me: Accepting Alzheimer's Without Losing Yourself* proves an Alzheimer's brain can continue to learn and flourish."

—Deborah Kan, executive editor and founder of *Being Patient*

"Love is by far the most used word in Rebecca Chopp's new book on living with Alzheimer's. Even today, five years since her diagnosis, Rebecca loves so much of her life: her painting, her hiking, her cherished husband, her dog. Rather than telling people to get their affairs in order, doctors should be required to give Rebecca's book to all new patients and to remind them that there is much life to live even after diagnosis. With erudition, love, and advice you can use on diet, mindfulness, and exercise, Rebecca provides a guidebook for *living* with Alzheimer's."

—Phil Gutis, former *New York Times* reporter
and columnist for *Being Patient*

"Ever the teacher, Rebecca Chopp provides brilliant instruction about how to remain happy, loving, and productive, even under the growing shadow of Alzheimer's. Ever the pastor, she draws from scripture, tradition, and her own remarkable life experiences to give us poignant lessons on how to abide with this illness and how to get and give help. Though Rebecca described herself as a 'brain attached to a body,' this book reveals the deeper reality that her family and friends have long known: she is a beautiful heart attached to a loving soul. *Still Me* is a profound, beautiful, and loving gift to the world to be long cherished and well used."

—John Witte, Jr., Robert W. Woodruff Professor of Law and McDonald Distinguished Professor of Religion, Emory University

Still Me

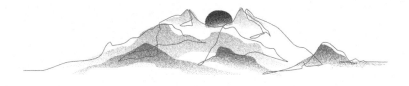

Still Me

*Accepting Alzheimer's Without
Losing Yourself*

REBECCA S. CHOPP, PhD

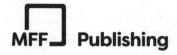

MFF Publishing

This book is intended as a reference volume only, not as a medical manual. The information given here is designed to help you make informed decisions about your health. It is not intended as a substitute for any treatment that may have been prescribed by your doctor. If you suspect that you have a medical problem, you should seek competent medical help. You should not begin a new health regimen without first consulting a medical professional.

Published by MFF Publishing
Denver, CO
morgridgefamilyfoundation.org/publishing/

The lyrics of the song "The Light" by Murray Deacock are included by permission of Murray Deacock, © 2023.

Except when otherwise noted, the subjects portrayed in the images in chapters seven and eight are unknown and were created by the author as an educational exercise.

Distributed by River Grove Books

Design and composition by Greenleaf Book Group and Kim Lance
Cover design by Greenleaf Book Group and Kim Lance
Cover image: Volha Kratkouskaya / iStock / Getty Images Plus

Publisher's Cataloging-in-Publication data is available.

Print ISBN: 979-8-9870082-4-9

eBook ISBN: 979-8-9870082-3-2

First Edition

TO FRED THIBODEAU

*My love, my friend, and my partner in
worldwide adventures.*

Contents

Contents

Me, Before and After

PRIOR TO MARCH 2019, people would describe me as a busy bee. From the time I was a young child, I was always on the go. I was known for being curious and imaginative, a mind with a body attached. I loved adventures, hiking, music. People who have known me as an adult describe me as being disciplined and scholarly. My professional reputation is that of a problem solver.

Now, going on five years after my Alzheimer's diagnosis, how would people describe me?

The same way.

Let me repeat that. The. Same. Way.

Maybe not *exactly* the same in the details. My hikes are now taken in the foothills near my home in Colorado instead of on mountains in far-flung places in the world. I now express my creativity through painting, a skill I began working on only after my diagnosis.

But everything that *was* me is *still* me. I'm still curious. Adventurous. Scholarly. I am still the most *Rebecca* when I am engaging in three areas of my life: the pursuit of justice and doing what is right; finding community with a shared and meaningful mission; and sharing time, love, trials, and triumphs with friends and family.

In some ways, this sameness surprises me—in part because in the meeting on March 6, 2019, where I learned of my Alzheimer's diagnosis, the neurologist told me that within two to three years I wouldn't be able to dress or feed myself.

She was wrong. But that meeting set me down a path of darkness. When I received the official diagnosis that cold and windy March day, I was filled with dread—a combination of desperate sadness and palpable fear. Not surprising given my family history of Alzheimer's.

A Family History of Alzheimer's

I have vivid memories from my childhood of my grandparents. They played a big part in our lives, as my parents didn't readily connect to civic or religious communities.

My paternal grandparents—Grandpa and Grandma Chopp, Frank and Gertie—lived on a farm in a Bohemian (Czech) community in the tiny town of Narka in northern Kansas. In Narka, even the store signs were in Czech. Grandpa Chopp was a large Eastern European man who wore coveralls, had enormous hands, and built fantasy houses for me out of straw bales. Grandma Chopp was a dumpling of a woman, round and smelling of bread and fried chicken. She seemed a bit crazy to me as a child, and I tended to keep my distance.

My maternal grandparents—Grandpa and Grandma McBratney— lived nearer to Salina. Grandpa Mac had been a farmer and a plumber and didn't talk much, preferring to watch TV and smoke his pipe. Grandma Mac was petite, like me, and full of energy. She was an avid smoker. A complicated woman fond of setting her daughters against one another, she was sophisticated, a bridge player, and a master gardener.

As a child, I spent a great deal of time playing and "farming" with Grandpa Chopp. When I grew older, and especially when I was in college, I'd spend hours talking with Grandma Mac. I fondly remember stopping by her small red house and sitting with her in her kitchen. She was even smaller than I and had a special "women's sewing" rocker that now sits in my home art studio. The oak rocker has a drawer underneath the seat where she would keep thread, needles, and her cigarettes. The kitchen was painted a sickening shade of green, and yellow linoleum chairs surrounded her table. I would sit at the table, she would sit in her rocker, next to a window filled with plants, and we would smoke and talk. She told me stories of her youth, especially stories of being an "Orphan Train" child.[1]

Both my grandmothers eventually suffered from dementia (as did my mother). Grandma Chopp, living in a rural county with little health care, lived in a nursing home for 15 years with a diagnosis of dementia. Grandma Mac developed Alzheimer's in her late 70s. She began losing more and more of her memory, forgetting to turn off the gas stove and leaving lit cigarettes on the table instead of in the ashtray. She had a small white-and-tan cocker spaniel/poodle mix, which I had given her. Over time, she struggled to remember to let the dog out. At the time, I was heading off to college and my mother still had my little brother to raise, so in-home care wasn't a practical option. So we moved Grandma Mac to a nursing home. Still, she found her way to the nurse's desk for her "smokes," since in those days they allowed smoking even in a nursing home. Gradually, she lost interest even in smoking and became, like my other grandmother had, totally bedridden, unable to recognize anyone.

I've never forgotten walking the halls of nursing homes where my grandmothers lived. It was mostly older women who were lined up in the hallways, their eyes blank, their hair uncombed, their clothes spattered with food. Some were tied to their chairs, their heads flopping, their mouths drooling, some not moving, some making motions with their hands. Occasionally I would see an older woman leading her Alzheimer's-afflicted husband around, while he looked helpless and hopeless, staring into nowhere. Those experiences with my grand-mothers' dementia were scarring.

Which is why it was those images that filled my mind when I received my diagnosis. Quite literally the stuff of nightmares. I felt like I was diving into Hell.

My family reacted much the same. How could they have any other reaction when facing the specter of what we all thought was my imminent decline and death?

One of the problems of Alzheimer's is the stigma that attends it: The images I just described are what most people think Alzheimer's looks like. They assume, explicitly or implicitly, that the diagnosis brings immediate and absolute failure.

I, too, had internalized this stigma. I thought only in binary terms: Either I had a healthy brain or I had a brain filled with wormholes. Either I was a fully functional adult or I could do nothing for myself. I was happy or I was empty. I was truly alive or I was as good as dead. As I came to learn, however, this binary mindset was far from the truth of Alzheimer's.

Learning to Live with Joy

Luckily, shortly after that initial diagnosis meeting, I switched to a different neurologist who had a quite different message for me. "Live with joy," she said.

In fact, the more I learned about this disease, the more I found that I could experience joy—that I could fight hard to stay well. In short, I learned that all hope had not and has not been lost. And from that point, my journey became one of doing everything I could to stay *me* for as long as I possibly could and not succumb to the Alzheimer's disease of my grandmothers. I frame the experience as struggling to stay in the light despite the darkness that is calling.

I've learned there is no one predictable path of Alzheimer's progression, though there are typical stages people progress through—each person in their own way and on their own timeline. Some go through the stages quickly, others more slowly. Some find they remain fully functional, save in one area such as reading or driving or handling math.

Many get an Alzheimer's diagnosis only when their symptoms are reaching the middle stages of the disease, which is typically when people are having trouble remembering the faces of loved ones or having difficulty finding their way around formerly familiar places. Many others will have my experience and receive a diagnosis early enough that they will have years *not only to live, but to live well.*

And there's the paradox. Though there is currently no cure in sight, the fight to live a fulfilling life in the face of an Alzheimer's diagnosis is not futile. Not unlike many forms of cancer, there are ways of fighting back. And, importantly, there's something worth fighting for. An Alzheimer's diagnosis is not a proclamation of imminent death. Those of us with the disease can live fully for many years. I want to say quickly that there is no sure-fire promise that any single step—doing more exercise, for example—will guarantee that you'll live longer and better. But there is mounting research to show a "brain healthy" lifestyle can help extend the good years.

I don't imagine that anyone will "skip" the sadness and fear associated with an Alzheimer's diagnosis, nor do I mean to suggest that I don't still feel moments of panic and desperation. Yet I work hard to live well and with joy. I am raising and training a puppy; I have discovered a latent passion for painting; I am writing this book; and I am making a new meaning of life—even as I know I am dying.

This isn't always easy. I tire easily, and even my focus for writing this book has been harder to maintain as the months have gone by from September 2022, when I first started writing, until I turned the manuscript over to the publisher in June 2023. I have bad days, and

I have to avoid a lot of activities that used to bring me joy. But for me, the fight means I will have more time with my family and friends, more time to give back to society, and more time to find new sources of joy and wonder.

I Want More Time

While I was writing this book, CMS (Medicare) announced plans to cover payments for FDA-approved drugs being used to slow the progress of Alzheimer's disease[2]—as I'll talk about in a later chapter. But the pace of progress in both research and Medicare in terms of support for Alzheimer's patients and treatments is still maddeningly slow. Not long ago, my son, sister, and I attended a rally at the Denver regional office of Medicare. I am an old lady with a significant and scary disease. But I have fight left in me. So there I was with my purple Alzheimer's T-shirt, against the backdrop of an American flag. Together, we marched. I carried a sign that said, simply, "I want more time."

Refuse to Surrender

As of now when I'm writing this book, there is no cure or even treatment with a high rate of success. But as I and other Alzheimer's advocates say, knowledge is power. What I know now is that this disease, when diagnosed early, can develop slowly. With the appropriate lifestyle treatment and with some of the promising new medications, the symptoms can show up more slowly. There are more and more instances of people living 20 years after an Alzheimer's diagnosis, though that is rare. Many of us with Alzheimer's go for years experiencing symptoms only as mild to moderate irritations.

The purpose of this book is to share my journey and what I have learned, in hopes that it may help others who have been diagnosed with Alzheimer's disease, Mild Cognitive Impairment (MCI), or other forms of dementia. I hope that I can inspire these patients and their caregivers to live with joy and to fight for their health as long as they can. I want others to find hope and make their way to living with good health and joy, even as they know they will eventually lose everything.

Though this book draws upon a great deal of research, I present all I have learned through my own story. You will follow me from my life before the diagnosis through almost five years of living with Alzheimer's. I want to tell those of you with Alzheimer's enough about me so you will understand my story and my choices—so you can hopefully apply the same processes to your own life, though obviously your choices will be different from mine. As I will say repeatedly, every person is different. How you respond will depend upon your history, your physical well-being, and your temperament.

My main message is that all of us need to refuse to surrender until we must! There are things we can do to help ourselves. We can extend our good days for ourselves and increase time with our loved ones. We can learn new ways to enjoy life and ways to give back to our communities. And who knows? Maybe a cure or better treatment will appear before the disease ravages our minds.

PART I

The Punch in the Gut

THANKS TO A LIFE that no working-class girl from Kansas could even imagine, I have had a memory-creating, abundant life. I was raised in a small town, then made my way to college, seminary, and graduate school. I am a wife, mother, minister, teacher, and theologian. Over the course of my professional career, I was fortunate enough to break gender barriers in the upper echelons of university administration.

By the time I was in my mid-60s, my husband, Fred Thibodeau, and I were living in a Denver, a city I have grown to love. I was the chancellor of the University of Denver, and had a 10-year plan that would lead to my retirement: finish out my administrative career, then afterward return to teaching. By then, according to my plan, I would be 75.

This final stop in Colorado also meant that my imagined retirement would include plenty of time with some of the people dearest to me, since the move had brought me closer to much of my family. My sister, Kathy Yeager, who is three years older than me and a stalwart friend, lived there. My son, Nate Biddle, and his wife, Lisa Hally, were also in Colorado. My younger brother, Tom Chopp, born when I was thirteen, and his wife, Colleen Warner Chopp, will eventually move to Colorado as well. I imagined, too, that I would have time to travel to visit close friends who live around the country and one in Peru. People, as you can tell, have been very important to me.

What's that saying about best-laid plans?

In the following chapters, I want to tell the story of how these plans came to a screeching halt.

1

The Lifetime of Memories I Will Lose

I AM GOING TO LOSE MYSELF, *for that is what a diagnosis of Alzheimer's means.*

The loss may not occur immediately and most certainly not all at once. But sooner or later, I will lose my "I"—my memories, my mind, and yes, my sanity. Saying I am filled with terror seems too mild.

Even before it happens, I regret losing my memories the most. Memories of holding my little boy and his sweet cuddles and his incredible energy, memories of his growing into adulthood, marrying and becoming a man. A memory of standing on the Yellow River in China at an archaeological dig. Memories of hikes in the Rockies, the Smokies, the White Mountains, and other places. The smell of the woods, the quiet of the forest, and the thrill of climbing up. Memories of Fred, who is so much more than a husband—a friend, my anchor, a playmate, a soul partner. Friends, places, food, experience. Every time I think about my Alzheimer's diagnosis, memories flood back, almost as though replaying those memories today might protect them from the inevitable.

Perhaps the first person who opened the door to this life of possibilities and of making memories was my first-grade teacher, Miss Roberts—a tall, thin woman who was always well dressed and infinitely kind.

I was shy, small for my age, with an unmistakable speech impediment. At one point, there had been discussion of institutionalizing me because tests could not measure intelligence in a child who could not speak. My mother—though she was not often my champion in life—insisted that I was smart enough for school and could understand what a teacher was saying.

Still, I was the butt of jokes by the other first graders and bullied on the playground. I would love to say "I will never forget Miss Roberts," who realized what a good reader I was and announced to the class that I would be grading everyone's spelling papers while the rest of the kids struggled to read aloud. But of course I *will* forget Miss Roberts.

I hate that I will lose my memories. So I treasure them now by remembering them on my walks, sketching them, by talking to them in my dreams. That's what this chapter is about—sharing those memories by way of documenting my life. I'll be going into more detail about some of these life experiences as they become relevant later in the book, but for now I just wanted to give you an understanding of how my life unfolded prior to receiving the Alzheimer's diagnosis.

A Farm Girl Goes to College

Born in the early 1950s in Salina, Kansas, I was a child of parents struggling to make it off the farms in northern Kansas. My father was a laborer and my mother a housewife.

My father was a moderately-sized man with dark skin and blue eyes who loved his children tremendously. He was an enormously kind and good man. He had little formal education and struggled with what I assume was a fairly severe learning disability, as he only learned to read when I was about eight years old. But he was driven and would eventually own several small businesses.

My mother, with fair skin and dark, wavy hair, was always overweight and lacking in self-confidence. She was one of the smartest people I have ever known, but she was always sad, depressed, and angry. She loved her children too, but she couldn't control her feelings of rage. Nor could she always keep her own self-confidence issues from turning into slights or insults against us. (My father died when he was 67 of lung cancer, and my mother died at 79 with Alzheimer's.)

Yet despite the precious memory of Miss Rogers and her faith in me, it took a long time for me to realize how smart I was. I didn't have a parent who told me "good job" or instilled confidence in my abilities. Teachers, by and large, ignored me because I was quiet and always did my work. My parents, creatures of their time and place, thought I might make a good housewife. They didn't go to college and saw no reason I should. So as a child, I prepared to be a homemaker. In high school, I was not enrolled in college preparatory classes; rather, I dreamed that I would meet a rancher and have seven children together.

It was only when my high school boyfriend got drafted to serve in the US Army during what was then called the "Vietnam Conflict" that I thought of continuing my education. When I started college against my parents' approval, I assumed that I would major in home economics or early childhood development.

I had wanted to see a bit of the world, and Kansas State University, 80 miles away from Salina, was a world quite different from my home. Too different, it turned out. I couldn't find an entrance ramp to the high-speed freeway. I didn't have the confidence to meet people, let alone seek out guidance. I didn't know how to study, and I had no idea I could ask for help. I would have been way too shy to go to a professor's office hours had I known they had them. I had the overwhelming sense that I didn't belong, and I couldn't seem to find friends or make connections with any clubs or groups. I floundered in that large state university and dropped out.

The one lesson I took with me when I left Kansas State happened this way: Before I gave up, one graduate assistant in a math course called me one day to ask me about my aspirations. I explained my dream of a ranch and seven children; by then I was dating a tall, handsome, and kind rancher named Larry, the man of my dreams. The grad assistant gently told me I was incredibly smart and should do something with the gift of my intellect. I laughed it off, as I knew I was in the midst of failing, but I heeded his advice and went back to college. I have long remembered his kindness.

Religion Major to Seminarian and Minister

I didn't realize it at first, but leaving the state university also meant leaving behind my dream of having a large family and living on a farm. Though not raised in a church home, I had always been keenly interested in religion and had a sense of connectedness to something greater, deeper, more ultimate than my world or myself. Since my home economics courses in high school were easy, I had plenty of free time to go to the town's library and check out books on various religions. I was fascinated. College and seminary ultimately provided me with a new language for these feelings and expanded my knowledge and understanding.

So when I switched to Kansas Wesleyan University, a college of 600 students in my hometown of Salina, I chose religion as a major. My professors opened doors for me to become a minister. Even while in college, I served two rural churches, Ashgrove and Barnard United Methodist Churches, not unusual in rural places where the supply of ministers was low.

After college I attended St. Paul School of Theology in Kansas City where I met and married my first husband, Mark Biddle, in 1974. In my third year of seminary, I had my son, Nate. After I graduated, Mark and I served Americus United Methodist in Americus, Kansas, as well as Calvary United Methodist in Emporia, Kansas.

In the early to mid '70s, most mainline Protestant churches weren't crazy about the idea of women ministers. My denomination was accepting but wasn't particularly supportive of having a married woman with a child as a minister, so I kept exploring other options. My seminary professors had urged me to get a PhD in theology, and in 1978, I took their advice and entered a program at the University of Chicago Divinity School. I was a duck out of water—one of the only women and the only person who had not attended a highly ranked undergraduate program. But I quickly jumped into that intellectually stimulating environment and stayed at U of C and taught several years.

In 1984, I went to Candler School of Theology at Emory University to teach in the seminary and in the PhD program. Mark and I sadly and with great regret ended our marriage in 1991, I think now because we grew apart after marrying so young. Several years after my divorce, I rediscovered my best friend from seminary, Fred Thibodeau, and we married in 1996. Fred and I remain a wonderful fit in values, styles, and sense of humor.

Academia Calls

Fred thought he was marrying a university professor and that we would have a nice, settled life in Atlanta. Out of nowhere, it seemed, I was asked to serve as interim provost at a university. The interim title was later lifted, and at age 45, I became provost of Emory University, a position I filled from 1996 to 2000. I really had no idea of what I was doing in this job, except that the president, Bill Chase, thought I could do the job. As provost, I was the most senior administrator after the president. I oversaw all the academic operations of the university, including the medical school, and was ultimately responsible for budget development across the university.

Along the way, I discovered that I loved administration: it combined my pastoral instincts and my love for teaching in ways that had an enormous impact. I loved the variety of people and projects as well as the occasional travel.

I went to Yale for a year, as a dean, and then decided I would pursue a presidency. I wanted to have more impact, and I wanted "my own thing." I then left Yale in 2001 to become the president of Colgate University, a position that, as I hoped, stretched me out of my comfort zone. I learned to lead, to build, to have fun at cocktail parties, and to be athletic. By that time, I knew my gifts had to do with developing a strategic plan for a school and raising money to execute that plan. I was good at making needed changes and also at moving a community forward. I did not enjoy maintaining a status quo.

After seven years at Colgate, in 2008 I became president at Swarthmore College, developed a strategic plan, and raised money. In 2014, I moved to the University of Denver to become its chancellor.

By way of preview for a theme that will arise later in this book, I'm sure that one of the reasons I gravitated toward senior administrative posts was to avoid having to take orders from others. When I was provost at Emory, the president empowered his three executive VPs to run their operations, set their strategy, and make their decisions. I learned so much from my colleagues, and we made a great team. After Emory I became dean of Yale Divinity School, one of the most distinguished theology programs in the world. The divinity school had multiple issues, many of them involving a complex building project that was under construction when I arrived. I collaborated with faculty and others to develop a strategic plan and ensure a bright future for this special school.

But, after a short while, I realized Yale and I were not a great fit. I didn't flourish within a large, tightly controlled university system that operated from the top down. This system was so different from Emory's collaborative culture, and it was not for me. Plus I had stepped from provost to dean and found myself in the middle of a system. I realized I was a better employer (CEO) than I was an employee. I did not like being in the middle. So after successfully straightening out the building project, at the end of the year I left to be the president of Colgate and never looked back. Few presidents in any sector serve as the CEO of three different institutions. I much prefer to be the one developing the culture, working with others to make decisions, and understanding that the final responsibility is on me.

A Mind with a Body Attached

On the journey that took me from rural Kansas to major universities, from farm fields to exotic locations around the globe, from a mind with a body attached to a mind waiting to lose its sense of self-awareness, I have come to develop a deep understanding of who I am as a person.

The graduate student at the large Kansas State University was perhaps the first person to point out that I was smart. Since that time, I have thought of myself as a mind with a body attached. It has been a running joke with friends, a constant source of "work" in therapy, and an incredible framework for my professional identity. I love learning; I enjoy entertaining myself with my mind.

I have made a living with my mind and found deep meaning in this life of the mind. I have written books and multiple articles. My mind was put to good use and was a bridge to connecting to new people in new ways. I loved nurturing seminary and graduate students as they learned new things and found new gifts. And I loved the play of ideas on a large university campus where I learned so many new perspectives and met people who were so passionate about their work.

As a higher education administrator, I delighted in setting strategies, supervising staff, solving problems, raising funds, building new facilities, and connecting my institutions to the world. My mind enabled me to educate thousands of young people and support research to make the world better. What a delightful life I led—a life of the mind that was beautiful, rich, and varied.

A beautiful mind. Perhaps that is why the thought of losing my mind is so frightening. And I will, bit by bit, lose it. I will lose my very identity and the mechanism through which I make my contributions to this world. I will become a body with a failing mind. I will not be able to solve problems or create new visions. I will lose the ability to entertain myself, to read, to paint, to dream.

But I have also come to appreciate or at least understand aspects of my temperament other than my intelligence. By temperament, I mean personality traits. The "busy bee" label I mentioned in the introduction was given to me by my family early in my childhood. I don't easily relax in an armchair or watch TV. I like to be active, and I have always needed my mind engaged. As a child, my favorite book was a series featuring a girl detective, Trixie Belden, who was curious, active, and never took no for an answer in her sleuthing. Those personality traits have inclined me to a life of learning and doing, which is one reason administration fits me well.

My personality traits have also led to a nearly absolute perfectionism, which I didn't begin to loosen until midlife. Since none of us can be perfect, perfectionism leads to a sense of failure and not being good enough. Some of my failures and inadequacies were real: I was not athletic and, despite my longings, I never made the cheerleading squad. I grew up believing I was an ugly duckling. I considered myself below average in most things and would have given myself a C minus as a human being. I think I inherited my mother's lack of self-confidence. But I was curious, active, and fueled by an enormous imagination.

Like my father, I am incredibly well disciplined, though I didn't realize this until I studied for my PhD, was married, raised a child, and worked—all at the same time. This discipline came in handy when I was a scholar and an administrator, and it helps me now with my rather intensive "living well" regime. Also like my father, I love deeply—though I am also a bit of an introvert, like my mother. In various roles as an administrator, my father's love of people came in handy. Now, in my earlier-than-planned retirement, with a diminished ability to handle crowds or even my favorite people for more than a few hours at a time, my mother's introversion serves me well.

As I have learned to see myself more clearly, I realized that I am practical and oriented to solving problems. I have my mother's creativity, though I typically drew upon mine when crafting visions for schools and now, much to my surprise, when I paint.

I have personality quirks quite my own. As an adult, I love adventure: hiking dangerous slopes or traveling to rural China, and now thinking of fun things to do like riding in a hot air balloon or going on a pilgrimage. My son was asked if he was surprised at how well I am doing in writing this book. He said, "No, my mother is very determined." I learned over the years to be determined if I needed to get something done. Ask some of the people who have worked for me over the years, and they'll tell you about my four a.m. emails and "do whatever it takes" approach to work.

I have an odd but ceaseless sense of humor, which is part of what helped me come out of my shell when meeting with alumni and donors. I am passionate about helping others. I tend to live out of my head and have had to learn to slow down and listen to others. Some of my worst mistakes as an administrator came from my tendency to solve problems and imagine opportunities on my own, rather than to slow down and consider what others had to say. I am stubborn and headstrong. These qualities are coming in surprisingly handy as I refuse to surrender before I have to.

The Fear of Madness

Perhaps it is ironic, given that I see myself as a mind with a body, but my greatest fear since I was a small child was that I would go insane, mad, crazy. This fear was later reinforced by my experiences dealing with my grandmothers' and mother's dementia, as I discussed in the introduction.

Unfortunately, there were other mental health issues in my family that fed into my fears. My mother suffered from severe depression, if not worse, and her angry and violent outbursts always frightened me. In rural Kansas in the 1950s and '60s there were no psychological resources or mental health counselors. Women who didn't fit the "happy housewife" expectations of the 1950s were often considered "a little crazy." Did my mother's madness become my worst fear? I don't know exactly when my fear started, but I was very young when the prison of madness came to dwell in visions.

As I grew older, the fear became more intense. I would hear of someone, often a teenager, committed to the Kansas State Mental Hospital and wonder when it would happen to me. In that era, mental illness was whispered about, often (mis)understood as a moral weakness or fault, and treated, in its extreme forms, by locking people away or giving them severe electric shocks. The insights and treatments we now have about mental illness were utterly absent from my world. All I knew about was insanity. Occasionally I watched movies where a person went insane. *One Flew Over the Cuckoo's Nest* was impossible for me to watch all the way through. And a semester of clinical pastoral education (where seminary students are trained in how to be present to those who are suffering) that included a rotation in a psych ward left me feeling I might end up in one of the beds.

My frequent nightmares were all about this vision of madness I so feared. In some, I went mad slowly, almost silently, until one day I woke up in a mental hospital of the old-fashioned kind, where "patients" were kept in straitjackets or chained to the walls. Sometimes I wasn't mad at all, but I was put in an insane asylum to be kept quiet because I knew too much or raised too many questions. Sometimes I would be fighting this imprisonment, or I would be drugged and unable to move. But my mind always returned to the knowledge that I was imprisoned.

The thought of madness—and all the images it invokes—makes me shudder to this day. I recently went to an art show in Taos, New Mexico. The work that grabbed me and held me was a small picture of a woman "gone mad." I don't know why I always feared this. Maybe it was the threat of being institutionalized as a young child because of my speech impediment. Maybe it was reading too much bad fiction in which women were committed to insane asylums.

Advocating for Mental Health

For much of my adult life, I have been an avid supporter of mental health. I did therapy with a wonderful woman and mentor who helped me integrate various parts of myself. I read avidly about mental health and various approaches to therapy and prevention. I became an activist in higher education and elsewhere to support mental health services. Of course, I learned that mental health is a spectrum, and the word insanity is a terrible, horrible word to be avoided. And yet in my nightmares, being "insane" still haunts me.

I am still scared to death of losing my sanity, and no matter how much I fine-tune my knowledge of what sanity is and as I learn more about what Alzheimer's does, I come back to this conclusion: I am, sooner or later, going to live my worst nightmare. The paradox of my life is that I am losing my sanity, my memories, my "I."

What I have to keep reminding myself is that I have a lot of life yet to live before I reach that point.

My Next Life Begins

I hope the biographical framework I've presented in this chapter will help you make sense of choices I've made as you read through the rest of the book and the factors that have shaped my perception of Alzheimer's disease. Whereas my old life story began at birth, my new life story begins with the Alzheimer's diagnosis, which I'll talk about in the next chapter.

2

Life, Interrupted

OCTOBER 12, 2018, STARTED OUT like any other day for me. As chancellor at the University of Denver (DU), my days were busy, intense, and always included a long list of things to do. I felt great, and I had a lot to accomplish.

By that October day, I was in my fifth year as chancellor of DU. My pre-retirement plan, as I mentioned earlier, was to serve as chancellor for another five years and then teach theology (my first professional love) for another several years. I was 67 and planned on having at least 10 good years of professional life ahead.

DU at the time was in the midst of realizing a bold strategic plan that I found exciting and motivating. I had developed a wonderful team of vice chancellors and was working with world-class faculty and staff. We needed to raise lots of money to provide financial aid, to build new buildings for our students and faculty, and to fund initiatives to engage and serve Denver, Colorado, and beyond.

I had just hired a firecracker provost, Jeremy Haefner, to be my partner in implementing our strategic plan and to work with the deans of our 10 graduate, professional, and undergraduate schools. I had just joined the board of trustees at Olin College, one of the country's top engineering schools.

I was fully engaged in university life in Denver and couldn't imagine any other place I'd rather be. Plus, I was delighted by the fact that for the first time in my adult life, I lived close to so many of my family members. I worked at least six days a week and had social events for DU and in Denver five nights a week.

Despite the demands of my job as chancellor—and the temptation to skip appointments relating to my personal well-being—I knew I had to take time to squeeze in an annual wellness exam. I was rarely sick, had never been admitted to a hospital, and had notably good health indicators. I worked out regularly, kept a healthy diet, and enjoyed a wonderful family life. Frankly, I had no reason to believe I needed to see the doctor. But I wanted to be healthy enough to enjoy my time at DU. So off I went that October day to see Dr. Jennifer McLean, who had been my trusted physician since 2014, when I arrived in Denver. That appointment changed the course of my life and laid the groundwork for my diagnosis of Alzheimer's, as I'll talk about in this chapter.

Lost in Denver

I typed the address of Dr. McLean's office into my GPS and set off. After about 20 minutes, I realized I had no idea where I was. I thought I was close, but I didn't know which way to turn. Frustrated and getting anxious about being late, I pulled into a parking lot of a bank and called my husband, Fred. Always on top of things, Fred called up his maps on the phone, figured out where I was, and directed me to the doctor's office. We laughed about the unusual occurrence. I had had a keen sense of direction all my life, but told myself that getting lost wasn't a problem because Dr. McLean had recently moved to a new office, and I had only been there once.

During the routine visit, the doctor asked how I was and whether I had noticed anything unusual. I told her there was just one thing, and it was very good news: I was sleeping eight to nine hours a night for the first time in my life! She knew my sleep history: I had never slept more than four to five hours per night (see sidebar). For most of my adult life, my nightly routine was to sleep from ten p.m. to midnight, get up and work for three or four hours, and return to sleep for a couple of hours (if I could). My mind never seemed to stop, and I loved using my mind to plan, solve problems, and draft documents in the middle of the night.

A Lifetime of Little Sleep

Even as a child, I routinely woke in the middle of the night. My father was often up working on his construction company's books or working on a new job proposal. I would take my dolls and my books and be content by his side for hours. I loved my father, and being next to him was one of the few moments I felt safe. My nighttime wakings became times of productivity and security. In graduate school, I would get up and study. My son was young, and I was juggling a job and a demanding graduate program. These extra hours each day came in handy. But it was not until I became an administrator that I realized this ability to get by on little sleep was a blessing—or so I thought. See chapter 15 for more on this topic.

I sometimes joked that needing so little sleep was my "secret sauce" since in a seven-day week I could actually put in nine days' worth of work (about 20 or so extra hours). For example, when I was the provost of Emory University, I quickly became friends with Dr. Michael Johns, the head of Emory Healthcare, who taught me a lot about being a senior administrator. But most of our "lessons" were conducted at two a.m. Michael didn't sleep much either, and we would work on the current set of problems and opportunities facing Emory. We had a lot of fun, and I learned a great deal.

Throughout my years at Emory, Yale, Colgate, Swarthmore, and DU, I followed the same pattern of sleeping little and getting much done.

Then, around March 2018—about seven months before my annual wellness exam and a year before the official Alzheimer's diagnosis—my sleep patterns changed dramatically. I started sleeping like a regular person. And I discovered I loved to sleep. Sleeping was fantastic, luxurious—like wallowing in a cloud or dancing in a field of flowers. I would wake fresh in the morning, run to the gym with new energy, and though I still drank coffee, I could stop at a cup or two instead of sipping away all day to stay caffeinated. On weekends, I discovered the magic of taking naps! Even as a child I couldn't fall asleep for naps and would lie still in agony, convincing my mother I was sleeping. No agony now—sleep was bliss.

Dr. McLean wrote this information down and asked me if there was anything else. I laughed and told her about getting lost on the way to her new office—such an unusual thing for me to do. She smiled slightly. Later in the exam, she asked me if I found reading or anything difficult. I told her not at all; I was proud of my ability to understand almost any printed material. I had been an effective speed reader since high school. Oh, I told her, there was one graph in the summer that for some reason I couldn't understand. It was a strange situation, and I brought it home to have my husband, who is gifted in math, help me. But that was all.

Nothing Is Simple

Near the end of my physical, the doctor asked if I would take a mini mental cognition exam. This time, it was my turn to smile. "Sure," I said.

The mini-exam took about 10 minutes and seemed simple enough. Simple questions, simple drawings, simple comprehension. I was confident I had aced it and would soon be on my way back to work.

But I hadn't aced it. Dr. McLean told me my results weren't quite what she had expected, and she wanted to refer me to a specialist to do more thorough testing. I agreed, believing that there must have been some odd fluke. I know enough about medical testing after years of supporting my parents and friends through various illnesses to never, ever be anxious about first results.

The specialist that Dr. McLean referred me to worked at the Kaiser Memory Care Center. When I called to set up an appointment, they informed me that Fred would need to attend as well. I thought that was totally unnecessary and quite inconvenient because the center was not close to home or work. But Fred and I drove off to a four-hour session filled with cognitive tests for me and interviews for both of us. I wasn't particularly nervous, just irritated by the interruption. Results would come some days later, but everyone I saw during the testing said, "You work too much; that's not good for your brain." I figured they said that to everyone they saw.

Several weeks later, we drove all the way back to the memory care center to get the results, which turned out to be all over the place: from "superior" to "below average," "mildly impaired," and even "moderately impaired." The interviews suggested some concern. More consultations and tests followed, and the experts at Kaiser said they needed more information, as they could not reach a conclusive diagnosis based on the mixed results from my testing. I was not sure what to make of this response, as Kaiser is a large system and has many neurologists, gerontologists, and other "memory care" experts. I figured whatever was going on, I needed to keep pursuing it.

Eventually, Kaiser referred me to an out-of-network expert neuropsychologist, Dr. Jay Schneiders, who specializes in complex cases. Suddenly, the status of my brain health seemed more serious.

Troubling Signs Ignored

Ever the researcher, I began to read about Mild Cognitive Impairment and Alzheimer's. Fred and I talked and talked about the past year. By the time I met with Dr. Schneiders, Fred and I were beginning to realize there were other troubling signs, things we had ignored or shrugged off.

First, I was having increasing difficulty remembering my daily appointments and relied almost completely upon the daily calendar card my assistant prepared for me. If I didn't check my electronic calendar on the weekend, I would often forget events or phone calls.

Second, whereas I had previously thrived on the social aspects of my administrative jobs, over the past year I had stopped wanting to attend social events, especially in the evening. In the morning, I would be excited about whatever event I was to attend that evening. I would plan out a special outfit and find myself daydreaming about taking some donors to the theater or stopping by a faculty reception after work. I loved the idea of going straight from work to a student gathering or just putting on my DU athletic wear and going to a basketball game. But by midafternoon I would be exhausted. The thought of being around anyone except Fred was more than I could bear. I just wanted to go home, sit for a bit, and sleep. I found myself canceling many plans and then feeling guilty for not doing that part of my job. Or I would ask the provost or someone else to fill in at the last minute for me. This had never been my habit in the past.

One event I remember skipping was the inaugural ball for Colorado's new governor, Jared Polis. I supported the new governor in his campaign, liked the vision he had for the state, and was wildly enthusiastic about the first gay governor and his partner having children. The ball was going to be relaxed, with lots of dancing. It sounded like a blast. I sent back the RSVP and began planning the "casual inaugural wear" the invitation requested. But about a week before the ball, I found myself dreading it. I knew it would be loud, long, and have way too many people for my comfort level. The dread grew, and I decided to ask the provost to attend instead. My mind supplied a great rationale: the provost was new; he needed to expand his connections in the state, and he and his wife needed to get on the Colorado social circuit. I put aside the dread and rationalized I was doing everyone a favor. I didn't give it any deeper thought, perhaps because my subconscious knew this change didn't bode well.

Third, I also found that I wasn't as organized as I once was. I was having trouble planning "next steps" in various projects.

As I developed a list of these and similar concerns, I began to think there might be a bit more of a problem than I had previously considered. I was nervous about the upcoming appointment, but I still thought that the "real" symptoms of MCI or Alzheimer's weren't showing up for me. Probably I was working too hard, as the Kaiser specialists had said. I started revising my timeline to step down as chancellor. Maybe I could transition to teaching after three more years instead of five. That was the state of my thinking prior to my meeting with Dr. Schneiders.

Reality Strikes

Dr. Schneiders spent a full day interviewing me and administering various tests. The conversations and results were a punch in the gut.

Dr. Schneiders was talking of a possible diagnosis of Mild Cognitive Impairment or early-stage Alzheimer's—the very conditions I had convinced myself I didn't have. Once again, just as at Kaiser, the results were all over the place, indicating everything from superior thinking to moderate impairment.

All my life, tests of any kind had been in the superior range. I had never tested below average or average in anything. Dr. Schneiders explained that thanks to my education and profession, I probably had lots of what he called "cognitive reserve"—which is the brain's ability to handle tasks in different ways—that helped me to function so well despite the changes going on in my brain. I had no idea what Dr. Schneiders meant by cognitive reserve (though I would later develop a deeper understanding, as I'll talk about in chapter 6). Indeed, I am not sure I could understand much of what he was saying. I was awash with emotions I couldn't name.

Dr. Schneiders was calm, relaxed, and radiated empathy. I am not a person who trusts easily, but I found myself wallowing in his kindness, in part to avoid the content of his words. In my life, failure (and I had failed these tests) had always been delivered with anger, disappointment, and accusation of fault. But Dr. Schneiders pointed no fingers. His care surrounded me like a soft, warm blanket. I left with the paradox of feeling his empathy while processing this potentially devastating news.

Because the results were so mixed, the investigation continued into what was occurring in my brain. On January 8, 2019, I had a positron emission tomography, or PET, scan done by the nuclear medicine department. This test is prescribed far too rarely due to its expense. The neurologists (and I met with several) all echoed what Dr. Schneiders had suggested: a diagnosis of MCI or possible early stages of Alzheimer's.

Each neurologist, psychologist, and social worker I saw said I needed to remove the stress of the job. Things were now serious. I was shocked, but I still didn't quite believe it.

Fred and I began to discuss how best we could get rid of the stress. Did we want to wait 10 more years before I fully retired? Was it safe for me to stay on as chancellor for another year or two to ensure a smooth transition? Fred, always attentive to planning around negative scenarios, began to look seriously at our financial situation. We ran through many "what if" scenarios. Still, my mindset was that at the end of all this, the diagnosis would be that I was experiencing very Mild Cognitive Impairment. Working a bit less would help improve my brain health.

Pretending Everything Is OK

The months between the initial wellness visit in October 2018 to early March 2019 were surreal as I continued with my very public job and, in the margins and cracks, tried to deal privately with the possible results of these tests.

I didn't—couldn't—breathe a word to anyone except Fred, my son and daughter-in-law, my sister, and my executive coach, Dick Nodell, that a problem might be emerging. I didn't want to cause any disruption or anxiety in a large institutional education system, and I knew that telling my close confidants would be difficult.

I got through the days pretending everything was OK. I desperately wanted to lose myself in the daily work of administration; in the engaging process of meeting with students, faculty, and others; and in keeping myself busy. All this work got me through the day but left me feeling even more exhausted at night, when I was even more anxious and fretful. In the middle of the night, the anxiety would erupt, interrupting that sleep I had recently come to enjoy and desperately needed. My nightmares about going mad returned, and Fred often had to wake me from struggling and screaming while I slept. I was beginning to feel like I was living two lives, and not quite sure which one was the most real.

During that period, I also came down with various illnesses. Migraine headaches started to interrupt my days. I once had to leave a senior staff retreat I was leading due to a migraine that was causing me to see flashes of bright lights. I caught every bug that went around. I ended up in the emergency room for the first time in my life with a severe bout of colitis. It was as if my body was screaming at me "Pay Attention: Something Is Wrong!" Or maybe the stress was working itself out physically because I didn't have much time to deal with things emotionally.

That was the state of my being prior to the official diagnosis of Alzheimer's, which I'll discuss in the next chapter.

Have You Been Ignoring Signs?

As I talked about in this chapter, only in retrospect did I realize I had shrugged off or ignored earlier signs that something was changing with my brain. So, I urge you to do what I didn't: Be honest with yourself about all the changes in your behavior, thinking, and capabilities. I'm not talking about one-time events, but rather changes in patterns (like my new fondness for sleeping) or the loss of abilities or talents (like my navigation skills) that are persistent or repeated.

3

No More Denial:
The Official Diagnosis

FINALLY, ON MARCH 6, 2019, I went to receive the diagnosis that would be entered into my medical record.

I dressed with care as if to signify to the doctors (and perhaps myself) that "I am sane." I wore my favorite St. John's knit jacket, checked with pink-and-white plaid. I had new black pants and my favorite black shoes. I brought a tote bag with all my records and a pad of paper. I projected the air of a prepared and capable student.

Inside, I was sick to my stomach. Fred was fidgeting but still, as always, comforting. We went to Kaiser's Franklin Center, parked on the highest level, and went to the fourth-floor neurology center. A woman sat with her husband in the right-hand corner of the waiting room. Her husband was hunched over, and his eyes were empty. She was wiping his nose. Across from this couple sat another man and wife. Her blouse was stained and not buttoned the right way; her hair was ratty, her hands restless. I whispered to my husband, "Don't ever let me look like that!" Whatever else might be coming my way, I couldn't stand the idea of looking like her. When the doctor called this couple, her husband helped her up, and she shuffled in.

There was now a pit in my stomach. I struggled to breathe deeply. It felt like I had been sentenced to a life of madness with the diagnosis of Alzheimer's that was upon me. And my body had known before my mind did. I didn't know at the time how devastating the upcoming meeting would be, nor the tenacity it would take to deal with the Alzheimer's diagnosis. Let me tell you how it all unfolded.

Warning! Lots of Science Jargon Ahead

In many ways, the process of getting an Alzheimer's diagnosis seemed designed to increase stress and confusion rather than the opposite. In this chapter, I've included just a sampling of the medical and biological terminology that was thrown at me, often without plain-English explanations. At times, it was difficult to understand exactly what the physicians were telling me and whether their diagnoses were the same or different. I've heard from many other Alzheimer's patients that they, too, have had to wade through technical jargon. Consider this a plea for practitioners to find simpler ways to communicate about complex issues like Alzheimer's.

How Not to Tell a Patient They Have Alzheimer's

When my name was called, I walked upright and with bright eyes into the doctor's office. Fred and I waited and waited for the doctor to arrive. We had met this doctor once before and found her somewhat dismissive and curt, yet knowledgeable.

Still, I could not have foreseen the inhumane interaction that was about to occur. I was about to learn the importance of finding a good fit with a neurologist.

The doctor began by bragging about how well trained she was—one of the top neurologists in the city and among the most rigorous. She dismissed my mother's Alzheimer's diagnosis as not relevant to me, saying it sounded like my mother had Lewy body dementia, and I showed no signs of that.

She had the 20-page report from Dr. Schneiders, who had made it clear he could only summarize his findings and not offer a medical diagnosis. His statement of results and observations read: "Neurocognitive disorder NOS—moderate severe; history of childhood onset speech and language disorder; mild MRI change in parietal lobe and cerebellar vermis; fatigue; hypersomnolence; adjustment d/o with mixed emotional features; personality change; apathy; decreased motivation." Of course, I didn't fully understand many of these terms at the time.

Further, this neurologist had made it clear that she was a "hard scientist" and put little store in what a psychologist like Dr. Schneiders said. So it was not clear whether she had read Dr. Schneiders's report at all; I wondered if she had simply skipped to his conclusion.

Based on all the information, including, in particular, the results from the PET scan that she had ordered, the reported diagnosis was "abnormal parietotemporal hypometabolism, findings which are consistent with the clinical concern of Alzheimer dementia." Once again, I didn't understand most of those words either, except for the part about dementia.

The doctor went on to say that I should stop working, and I should start telling people I was in the early stages of Alzheimer's. When my husband asked her what we should expect, she said that in two to three years I probably wouldn't be able to button my clothes, let alone drive or do other basic tasks.

If I weren't so good at being composed, I might have fallen out of my chair in shock or slugged her for her tone. We were ushered out.

What happened to me should not happen to anyone. Maybe that doctor was having a bad day. Maybe she had been hardened by too many sad cases before mine. But the way the news was shared and the images she planted in my brain were entirely unnecessary.

Back in the car, Fred and I cried—angry at her treatment of us, frightened by the diagnosis, and utterly confused by hearing the neurologist say "MCI" and "Alzheimer's" in the same sentence.

I could only see images of myself slobbering, incoherent, unbuttoned. In just a couple of years, I would be as disheveled and empty-eyed as the woman I had seen in the waiting room.

I am extremely independent and couldn't bear the thought of even my husband taking care of me. No, no, no!

I called into the office and said I was sick. We went home to process.

Major Life Decisions

Because of the timing of the academic year and an upcoming board meeting, I knew I was going to have to make some tough decisions about staying on as chancellor.

In truth, Fred and I both knew what the decision was going to be: I needed to retire. Since our first trip to the memory care unit, every doctor had said I worked too hard. All of our research pointed to the fact that stress would only accelerate the progress of the disease. And there was no way to stay at the helm of a complex university and avoid stress. I wanted to spend time with my family and use whatever "good time" I might have left to enjoy life.

The question became *when* I would retire and how I would explain it. Should I retire in two years or a year? Could I make it? Should I retire abruptly on July 1, at the end of the academic year? I was pulled in two directions. I didn't want to risk hurting DU. But that is complicated.

Stepping down immediately would be a shock to the institutional system and a blow to my staff, my board, and my many friends. But if my disease progressed rapidly, I might make a mistake that could be costly to the institution or hurtful to good people.

On the other hand, I knew that the first diagnosis of rapid slide into the moderate stages of Alzheimer's might turn out to be true. What if I only had two or three years, even under the best circumstances of no stress and healthy living, before I started turning into a vegetable—before the madness descended?

For 25 years, Fred had never complained about my working day and night. He loved being with me and still put up with my constant travels around the world. But now, with the shadow of Alzheimer's looming, I wanted to spend more time with him. And with my son, Nate, who lives near me; I love doing things with him and his wife, Lisa. My sister and I have been close since we were little girls and enjoy hiking, working out, and all sorts of other activities. I am a person who adores my close friends—and have always looked forward to more time with them in retirement.

Finally, I realized there was a possible alternative. Jeremy, the new provost and executive vice chancellor I had recently hired, might become an interim chancellor. Provosts often move into presidencies and almost always serve as an interim in an emergency. I proposed to Jeremy that I suggest to the board of trustees that he serve as interim chancellor, giving the board time to figure out if they wanted to conduct a search for the new chancellor or appoint him fully. He agreed.

I had a tentative plan, subject to the approval of the board of trustees, for how the university could have continuity of leadership. But what about me? I needed to find a new neurologist, and, scariest of all, I needed to figure out how to explain my resignation.

Finding a Doctor That Fit

I am a trained researcher, and my husband is very fact-oriented. We spent a lot of time researching MCI and Alzheimer's. Eighty percent of those diagnosed with MCI develop Alzheimer's. And some physicians do not want to give the diagnosis of Alzheimer's until symptoms usually associated with the moderate stages of the disease begin to show. Based on what we gathered, we started to understand the previous neurologist's diagnosis. Notwithstanding her off-putting assurances that she was essentially one of the brightest in the land, we didn't doubt her competence.

Still, we needed more of an explanation about what was going on in my brain. I wanted a second opinion and decided to go out of my Kaiser insurance network for it.

This next doctor was very caring, which I quickly discovered both Fred and I needed. She read all the reports carefully and asked many questions about the progression of my mother's disease, my childhood speech impediment, my own feelings, and the perceptions of my husband. She showed us the PET scan images and explained where the issues were in the brain, including the fact that there might have been an early wound in the brain that caused the onset of the speech impediment. She explained in great detail the meaning of Dr. Schneiders's test and noted he was one of the most competent neuropsychologists in the country.

This doctor confirmed I had MCI and, most likely, Alzheimer's. She was caring, wise, comforting, and full of information. She took a full hour and offered to talk again anytime, even by email or phone. If paying for an out-of-network neurologist weren't cost prohibitive, I would have signed up with her on the spot.

Going forward, Fred and I knew we would need a caring as well as rigorous doctor. Our primary care physician suggested I make an appointment with Dr. Lynsee Hudson. She was in network, but we could not get an appointment with her until a month later, on April 17.

When I met with Dr. Hudson, I knew she was the right fit for me. What a gift she was! Warm, friendly, extremely knowledgeable, and upbeat. From the moment I met Dr. Hudson, I knew she was going to encourage us, even as she helped us to confront a difficult reality. She had reviewed all the tests and all the neurologists' reports so far. She included Fred fully into the conversation, but was also speaking directly to me. Dr. Hudson's basic diagnosis read: "Cognitive dysfunction in the range of MCI but with radiographic and clinical features (PET/MRI) supportive of pattern of Alzheimer's, with her high premorbid IQ I do believe she has fairly significant cognitive loss despite residual high functional status and good performance." While I came to understand that Dr. Hudson's diagnosis was essentially the same as that of the previous neurologist, the way she delivered the message made all the difference in my comprehension and comfort level.

From the Physician's Viewpoint

I have a lot of sympathy for neurologists who work with Alzheimer's and other patients with permanent brain deficits. Most or maybe all the people who become doctors want to make people better. Though I do believe there are ways that doctors can help people live wonderful lives even with an Alzheimer's diagnosis, it must be frustrating to them that there is no way, as of yet, to cure this disease, and the progress is sad and painful.

After months of struggling with all the hypotheticals and developing tentative plans, it was oddly comforting to get a formal and clear diagnosis from a doctor I knew was being realistic and compassionate.

Then Dr. Hudson turned to the issues of what to do now. I told her my tentative plan to step down as chancellor, and she agreed that was necessary for my health. But she also said she wanted me to live well: to take care of myself, to find joy, to exercise and dance, to do art and express myself, to have social engagement, and to continue to be intellectually engaged. She used the most amazing phrase: "Live with joy."

Frankly, I hadn't even thought about the immediate future beyond my early retirement but before the inevitable descent. Joy? Live well? Dance? Who talks like this when they hand out an Alzheimer's diagnosis?

Processing the Raw Fear

As we walked from Dr. Hudson's office, Fred and I began to truly accept the diagnosis that I had Alzheimer's. The raw fear enveloped me, but I made it to the car before I broke down in convulsive tears. I am not a person who cries much, but there was no way to stop the tears. Alzheimer's was now in my medical record, and I was really and truly going to lose my mind, to forget even my closest loved ones' names—to go mad, just as I had always feared.

I was still shaking when we got back to our downtown condo building. No one joined us in the elevator, thank God. We made it inside and held each other. And we cried and cried. Despite six months of all the what-ifs, despite having a mother and both grandmothers who had died from Alzheimer's, despite reading everything we could to prepare for this moment, we were totally shocked. We cried off and on all afternoon.

Fred and I had a favorite restaurant catty-corner from our condo. Blue Agave Grill was often the place we went to relax, talk, celebrate, and sometimes to be frustrated with my work or his volunteer activity serving on the board of the condo association. We had "our" booth in the back corner where we almost always sat. That evening, the server took one look at us and took us to the corner. We cried, drank margaritas, and (I suppose) ate. Neither of us tended to drink much, and Fred hardly ever had even a single drink. But that night, I remember Fred was a bit wobbly on the way home. Drowning our sorrows in alcohol may not have been the healthiest response, but it was how we coped that night.

I called in sick to my office the next day. We had to make some immediate plans.

One of the hardest parts of processing the diagnosis was the challenge to the very essence of my being. No one has ever described me as needy. I do things for myself and take care of myself. It is the deepest personal code I have. It is my survival mechanism and my joy. My favorite T-shirt says "Tell Me What You Think I Can't Do So I Can Get Started." I remember the exasperation of my father teaching me to ride my first bike, when I kept saying, "Hands off, I can do it!" The beautiful light blue bike and I would fall. He would say gently, "Let me help you." My response was always, "No, Daddy, I can do it."

Yet now, six decades later, this independence would be lost. I would (soon, I thought) not be able to feed myself, pick out my clothes, make it to the bathroom by myself, or even remember to shower.

Every cell in my body screamed NO, NO, NO! I did not want my loved ones to feed me or bathe me. I didn't want caretakers to dress me. I thought about how Fred would probably dress me in beige (his favorite color), and I begged my sister to make sure I had plenty of clothes in orange, purple, and magenta. I wished I were in a culture where elders were expected to go to a mountaintop and give themselves to the gods.

I looked at the mountains around me and wondered if I was brave enough to do that. The alternative seemed far more bleak.

A Bad Year Gets Worse

During this same period, in late March 2019, we learned that my husband's eldest son, Matt Thibodeau, would have to have a heart transplant if they could find a suitable heart. Matt was only 44 at the time but had worn a pacemaker since he was in his mid-30s. His heart had deteriorated in recent years. When we flew to San Francisco in early April, we were scared for Matt. But we had no idea what bad shape he was in until we saw him. To make it worse, the hospital was finding it difficult to find a suitable heart. He was placed on a left ventricular assist device to keep his blood pumping and was receiving kidney dialysis.

Fred was terrified—filled with grief and anxiety. I was trying to support my husband, while worrying about Matt and still trying to process my own news. Still unable to find a suitable heart, the doctors told us that time was running out quickly. Then, in the middle of the night, on April 4, Fred got a call. They had found a heart and moved into emergency surgery. Matt recovered slowly, as the damage to his body was significant. He was in the intensive care unit for six weeks, much longer than people twice his age usually needed. But he did recover after weeks in the hospital and months of care at home. Fred flew out frequently, coming back to Denver to be with me (including when I told the DU board my news, which I'll discuss in the next chapter).

Navigating both of these terrifying events at once was, for me, like being on the edge of a flat earth, pulled in so many directions. I wanted to support my husband, of course, as he dealt with his son's immediate life-and-death situation. But I was facing the most difficult moment of my professional career—telling a board and others I had to resign and then making a public announcement. So much for trying to avoid stress!

Information Is Power

As you've seen in my story, diagnosing Alzheimer's is a process, in my case taking six months. It can involve multiple tests and scans and consultations with many different doctors, nurses, technicians, and specialists. Communication between all the people involved can fail, records can be lost, and everything takes way too long. I often wondered how those not familiar with complex bureaucracies could navigate it all. I found it difficult, and I was used to complex institutions in my own career.

Receiving the diagnosis of Alzheimer's is not easy, but it is absolutely imperative if you want to fight back against the disease. I have told the story of my diagnosis, in part as a way to encourage others to get diagnosed early. The earlier the diagnosis, the sooner you can intervene. And the sooner you can begin to deal with the inevitable shock and despair, the longer you can enjoy the light.

My diagnosis was unusual, as I wasn't aware of symptoms, though I now realize I was starting to show some. But soon—and much earlier than I would have liked—there came a time when I could no longer put off the inevitable. Having a clear diagnosis of Alzheimer's meant I needed to figure out how to share the news with family and friends, the DU board, and the public, and to step down from the position I had enjoyed for so many years. That's what I'll talk about in the next chapter.

Find a Neurologist You're Comfortable With

I learned a valuable lesson in comparing how I was treated by the first neurologist who gave an official diagnosis of MCI and how subsequent physicians treated me: **Do what you can to find a neurologist who is a good fit for you.** I was fortunate that Dr. Hudson, the neurologist I finally found, not only told me to live with joy, but also gave me tools to learn to do so.

Finding a doctor you feel comfortable with isn't an easy task, as there are not enough neurologists to address the current need, and navigating insurance coverage and health-care systems can easily become overwhelming. All I can advise you to do is persevere. Don't settle for medical care you think is lacking in any way.

4

From the Fast Lane to the Parking Lot

AS OF JULY 1, 2019, I WAS RETIRED. Suddenly "free" of all the responsibility and stress of running a university, I was awash in all my losses. I sobbed, thinking about the fact that I would never again help first-year students move into their dorms, greet new faculty members, or confer degrees at commencement. I wouldn't create strategic plans, build buildings, or raise money for scholarships. It felt odd to no longer be "the chancellor" or even Professor Rebecca. I had looked forward to all those daily interactions with staff and with people across campus and in Denver. The daily fabric of my life vanished instantly. How I spent my days—what I thought about morning, noon, and night, how and where I had built so much of my identity—was now in the past.

In this chapter, I'll talk about the buildup to that fateful day, which was a challenging and painful period as the news of my diagnosis spread. It's wasn't easy then and still isn't easy to face the new realities of my life.

Private News Made Public

My first priority in terms of dealing with the professional consequences of my diagnosis was to share the news with the DU board chair, Denise

O'Leary. I emailed Denise the day after I had the appointment with Dr. Hudson, and told her there was something urgent to discuss. She responded by inviting me to her house for lunch a few days later. I was relieved not to have to tell her over the phone or in my office.

Over the intervening days, I began to process how to share the news. I knew I would tell my family and close friends that I had been diagnosed with Alzheimer's, but several professionals had advised me to think carefully about what I shared publicly. Why? Because, in their experience, people often reacted negatively to the diagnosis of Alzheimer's, given the tremendous stigma the disease carries with it. Out of fear and ignorance, people tend to back away quickly—as I would soon discover firsthand. Some seem to think a person with such a diagnosis is unreachable—as though one immediately becomes incompetent upon diagnosis. Others might find it scary to be around someone with this disease, perhaps because they "don't know what to say" or don't want to think much about something so difficult. It's often easier to help someone with other kinds of terminal disease, I was told; you can't tell someone with Alzheimer's to "get well soon."

So I made calls to some of my most trusted professional colleagues to get their advice on what to say publicly. As a chancellor of a well-known university, and having had a 25-year career in the national landscape of higher education, people would want to know *why* I was stepping down on short notice. I was going to need to develop a narrative quickly.

I drove to Denise's house for our scheduled lunch. I was a nervous wreck but thought I acted fine. Yet Denise could sense immediately that something was wrong. We fixed our lunch and went to her back porch, sitting in chairs facing the mountains. It was a beautiful spring day. She showed me the owls' nest in her yard, and we admired how much snow was still on the mountains. Then her piercing eyes turned to me. "Well, what's up, Rebecca? What's going on?" As I gently wept,

I told her my diagnosis and about the last seven months of tests. I don't remember exactly what she said; all I knew was we were holding hands and sobbing together.

I swallowed hard and told her that Fred and I had decided I needed to step down as chancellor as soon as possible. I told her I would stay through the end of the academic year.

Sharing the News More Widely

I turned to family and friends for support. Fred and I had kept my son, Nate, and his wife, Lisa, abreast of the tests. Nate and I are very close, and the four of us enjoy living near each other. Although much is written about an adult child learning of a parent's diagnosis, little is written about how an adult parent feels when telling a child she has Alzheimer's. A parent wants to protect a child, no matter their age. I always felt it was my son's role to come to me for help, and now I would, sooner or later, need his help.

We sat at the dining room table where we often sat for holiday feasts or simple Sunday lunches. I don't recall if it was Fred or I who confirmed the news that I had been diagnosed with Alzheimer's. Nate and I cried a little, but the conversation quickly turned to his and Lisa's pledge of support. They promised to do whatever they could to help. Nate had already been reading about Alzheimer's, and we discussed behavioral interventions as well as various treatments. Next, I had to tell my sister and brother and my closest friends.

As I told friends, and began to work with Denise and a few others, I had to figure out what I was going to say. I knew that I would tell close friends and the DU board that I had been diagnosed with early-stage Alzheimer's. But I was not sure I was ready to announce that to the world. I was scared of the stigma and didn't want everyone treating me as if I were further along the progression of the disease than I was or avoiding me from fear that they could somehow could catch it! I don't like to think of myself as the subject of gossip, and I hated the picture of people wondering whether this or that decision I had made as chancellor was affected by my condition. I was still trying to learn all I could about the disease and wasn't ready for all the questions I might get. And, most importantly, I was not ready emotionally to announce it to the world.

I imagined a headline in the *Denver Post* with my name and the word Alzheimer's, and it all seemed too much. After consulting with some of my closest colleagues, I decided to announce that I had been diagnosed with a "complex neurological disorder" and that I needed to step down as chancellor.

In early May 2019, it was time to tell the board of trustees. A hush fell over the room as I shared the news of my diagnosis and imminent retirement. Finally one board member, crying, spoke of his fondness for me, of his respect for me, and of his support for me. In what I can only describe as an experience of heavenly grace, one by one each board member spoke. To my amazement, nearly everyone in the room cried. The expressions of love and affection filled my soul. Several of the board members were investors in Alzheimer's research or had connections with the best research centers in the country. Each one offered to help.

The public announcement followed. Because I was not yet ready to announce my specific diagnosis to the general public, I kept the announcement short and factual: that doctors had "diagnosed me with a complex neurological disorder that I need to attend to sooner rather than later" and therefore I would resign from my position as chancellor at the end of the academic year (June 30). And then I asked the community for privacy: "I would request that you not ask for further details about my health at this time. We need privacy in order to move forward and make sense of this unexpected turn of events."

The Transition to Chancellor Emerita

At my final commencement, after presiding over 21 such ceremonies, I simply wanted to make it through the events. DU holds its graduate commencement on a Friday evening and its undergraduate commencement the following morning. I wasn't surprised when especially so many of the social workers, psychologists, humanists, and educators, as well as others graduating Friday night, hugged me and wished me well. But I was totally surprised the next morning by the undergraduates.

In the DU culture, the college graduation ceremony is all about those students; that day is *their* special day. I didn't want or expect them to be thinking about anything but their own accomplishments and their thanks for faculty, family, and friends who had helped them. I was shocked when so many of them wanted to hug me, tell me they would pray for me, say thank you for all I did, and generally show me their love. DU has approximately 6,000 undergraduates, and I only got to meet a small fraction of them individually during their time as students. So this stunning display of affection and grace was an unexpectedly beautiful conclusion to my lifelong goal to help students do well and do good by contributing to society and making the world a better place.

Look for Signs of Grace

This terrifying journey for me has been alleviated in small ways by moments such as what happened in the board meeting and at that last graduation ceremony: signs of grace in and through community—entirely unexpected, but always deeply appreciated and held on to in my memory as long as I keep it.

With that done, as of July 1, 2019, I became chancellor emerita—an honorary title that I cherish, but one that comes with no job responsibilities. Though I was to be involved in a few projects at DU for the next year or so, I had to radically invent a new life for myself while getting my mind around having a terminal disease.

All my career I had moved from one position to another. A common family joke when retirement would come up was "Rebecca will never retire." I always had to be busy. Once I was old enough to work, I filled my time with various jobs. When I discovered ways to combine my passion of mind with work in teaching, research, and higher education, I was happy, engaged, and busy. I don't believe I was running from anything; my mind and body just liked to live in the fast lane. While I almost always missed people from the places I left, I always felt excited about who I would meet next and what we would accomplish together. And now, it seemed, there was nothing to look forward to.

So many of the retirees I have known over the years have struggled with how to fill their newly unstructured time. I think part of my fear of going insane is not having enough to do. The few times I have been bored in my life, I felt on the edge of madness. As I've said, I had never worried about having an empty schedule because I had my plan of serving as chancellor for five more years before transitioning back into teaching, and then retiring to write a book or two about teaching and maybe one in theology.

So what the heck was I going to do now that I had moved from the fast lane to what felt like the parking lot? What was I going to become—or, perhaps, what was going to become of me?

The University of Denver was gracious enough to give me a part-time consulting role. I chaired a search committee hiring a new vice chancellor and served on another committee or two. I even had an office at DU for that first year of being the chancellor emerita. The office was in this high tower accessible only by an elevator installed in 1918. In this single room with no other staff members, I enjoyed a gorgeous view of the mountains, but the thin windows meant that the office was uncomfortably cold in the winter, reminding me of how isolated I was—literally alone in a tower. That office struck me as a metaphor for my current life: isolated, cold, far removed from my rich and wonderful life, which until recently I had lived just floors below me in the same building.

I was fearful I would drive my husband, who had been retired for about 10 years, out of his mind. Fred is grounded and entertains himself well. He doesn't need a lot of rush and bustle in his life. He reads a great deal and tracks all sorts of sports statistics. Would I be like so many spouses who retire and drive the other spouse wild? I remember my father retiring, being bored, and deciding he wanted to redecorate the house, which, until then, had been completely my mother's domain. His puttering around, his being underfoot, his wanting to change the rules and the visual space created intense anxiety.

I didn't have many hobbies outside of my exercise routines. But hiking is an occasional event, and working out only fills a small portion of the day. I never took to cards or puzzles or golf or other things people often enjoy in their retirement.

Slipping Away

Awhile ago, I began to realize that even when I intended to do something—even when I wrote notes to myself, talked to others about what I was going to do, and thought about it for several days—I would still forget to do it. Sometimes even seemingly trivial situations hit hard.

In 2022, I volunteered to cook the turkey for our Thanksgiving feast. I find turkey often dry and way too bland, but it is a tradition, and others in my family love the traditional turkey, stuffing, and cranberry sauce. Several years ago, I had heard that cooking the turkey breast-side down with the legs up in the air results in a juicer bird. What the heck? This might be the last time I cooked a big bird, so I decided to experiment. I read many online recipes and talked to my son, who had cooked his turkey this way many times. I even compared notes with my neighbors on turkey cooking methods, and I told my husband to make sure I baked it this way. I may have Alzheimer's, but after 40-plus years of cooking turkey one way, I was trying something different! I woke up at five thirty on Thanksgiving morning, put the dry rub on the turkey, and set out the big bird to let it come closer to room temperature. I returned home from an hour's walk and popped the turkey into the hot oven. I didn't baste it or open the door per all the recipes I had read and the expert advice of my son. Five hours later, when my son, who was carving the turkey, pulled the bird out, it was breast-side up. He said, "Oh Mom, you decided not to cook it breast-side down?"

I was chagrined, shocked, and quite frankly, furious at myself. How had that happened? And what the heck was happening to me? I used to remember the details of a complex university budget. I often remembered details of legal cases better than our lawyers did. I could recall complex and long lectures in theology or presentations on the state of the university. And now, I couldn't remember to turn over a big dead bird. I was deeply embarrassed over this seemingly silly mistake.

Can I Stop the Slide into Darkness?

It struck me at one point that I wasn't simply retired, I had been *forced* to retire because of my Alzheimer's diagnosis. I had received a death sentence. I saw Alzheimer's as a slow (or maybe even fast?) road to losing my mind. And I was terrified.

Now that I was retired, I had seemingly infinite time to sink into my emotions. It may sound corny, but dread's darkness and coldness settled into my soul. In other dark times in my life, when I faced a challenge or awful situation, I had eventually found a way to escape. The worst time for me came the year after my divorce. I was in my mid-30s. I lost a year to a deep depression—sometimes unable to move, drinking too much, avoiding suicide only because I loved my son too much to leave him. I was empty. I was in the pit of desolation. I thought I had cried out all my tears of failure, loss, and devastation that year. But even then, I had my love for my son (who was having his own difficult time) and an incredible therapist who helped me to see, ever so slowly, that I had a future. The heavy darkness of severe depression began to lighten. Eventually, through a long struggle, lots of therapy, and time to heal from the divorce, I began to feel tinges and tingles of hope again.

But this time, I saw no way out. No cause for hope. I sensed a profound darkness around losing my memories, my mind, my sanity. A frigid coldness around not knowing my family, what to wear, where I was. I started reading some stories of those with Alzheimer's, which reinforced my worst nightmares that I discussed earlier: sitting and staring blankly into space. I heard about Alzheimer's patients wandering into the night. A man in our condo building pushed his wife, a victim of Alzheimer's, around to meetings and events as she slumped, largely unresponsive, in her wheelchair.

At the time, I was unaware of any counterexamples—of people living and thriving after their diagnosis.

Dark times, indeed. I can't imagine that anyone who receives an Alzheimer's diagnosis won't have them. But fortunately, I came to realize that I had strengths and abilities that could help me fight to achieve a joyful life, as Dr. Hudson had recommended. How I reached that point is the subject of Part II.

Tips for You

Knowing you have Alzheimer's can feel very isolating. Don't let that happen. Try to avoid withdrawing from the things that make you happy. Reach out to the people you trust to get advice on how and when to share the news and what messages to share with which people or groups.

PART II

Aftermath

NO MATTER HOW THE NEWS IS DELIVERED, the shock of an Alzheimer's diagnosis cannot be minimized. Your entire world changes. Getting a diagnosis of any terrible disease is devastating. But whereas so many other diseases have at least a chance of a cure, there is no cure for this one.

It was in those first months after the diagnosis that the fears I've mentioned before became nearly all-consuming. All I could think about, at first, was my once active grandmother Mac in her final days, trapped in her chair, vacant eyes that seemed to see only darkness, maybe a few shadows. The most vibrant person I knew in my childhood now seemed among the living dead—there, but only in body.

I thought about my mother's hallucinations as she suffered with dementia. I recalled my other grandmother, confined to her bed in a nursing home for years. I saw the shuffling patients with their dirty clothes and unkempt hair at my neurologist's office.

Worst of all, because of the fear and misinformation, some from that first neurologist, I could not see these inevitabilities as distant. No, they felt imminent. Like one day soon I would be lost. As though tomorrow morning, I might not recognize Fred—might look in the mirror and see a confused ghost looking back at me.

As I lamented all that I would lose, depression seemed to be taking over my life. I imagine this is where many people start to give up, whether or not they realize it. I felt that temptation. I had been forced to walk away from the life and identity I had come to know. I didn't want to leave my house. The prospect was daunting—not because I saw signs of decline, but because I knew that decline was inevitable. Rather than call my sister and go for a hike, I found myself sitting at home, wondering how much longer I'd even be able to hike. Seeing my son was painful: all I could think about was how I would lose him and how he would be left with a shell of a mother. In a word, it all felt hopeless.

While I was in this turmoil, I kept thinking about the advice Dr. Hudson had given me in her prescription to live with joy. Deep down, I also knew I had to do something. I owed it to my family, and I didn't want to just sit and despair until my symptoms worsened. Whether it be three years or ten, I owed it to myself and everyone around me to not surrender yet.

It was hard at first to listen to that part of myself—the part that was whispering "fight back; it's not over yet." But I listened hard to that whisper and allowed myself to hear it more clearly. I knew from my own experience and from watching too many friends, congregants, students, and colleagues suffer so many tragic losses that in the midst of that despair, one can still take action to lighten the darkness. How I found that inspiration is the subject of the following chapters.

5

Lightening the Darkness
of Despair

I THINK IT WILL COME AS no surprise that my initial reaction after receiving the diagnosis was that I had been consigned to Hell.

Hell, in some Christian expressions, is the place bad people are condemned to burn for their sins. Hell doesn't fit with my image of a loving and redeeming God. I don't believe in Hell; it just isn't there in my spiritual imagination and soul. But I found myself thinking about Hades of Greek mythology. Hades is the god of the underworld that bears his name: a place of coldness and darkness, of wandering in the mist. Hades came to represent *my* underworld, the underbelly of life I might never completely be able to leave.

But did I have to stay in this misty, cold underworld *all* the time? Could I find a way to combine the darkness and dread of Hades with the joy and wellness of living in the light, even if it was increasingly cloudy?

A good friend helped me answer that question by reminding me of another aspect of the Hades mythology, the story of Persephone. She was the daughter of Demeter, goddess of the harvest. Persephone was the maiden who helped her mother give life to all plants. She was creative, full of life and joy. Her special role was bringing all the colors to the flowers, which in turn attract the bees to pollinate the plants. According to the myth, the people of the earth depended upon the work of Demeter and Persephone to grow their crops and provide natural beauty in the world.

One day Persephone saw the most beautiful flower, a dark red-black orchid, and ran across the fields to see it. That attracted the attention of Hades, the god of the underworld, who snatched her to be his wife. Persephone suddenly found herself no longer in the light, no longer surrounded by color and warmth, but in the cold, dark underworld, where earth's beings went after they died. Thanks to the help of Styx, the goddess of the river between life and death, Persephone began to see through the mist. She started to draw again and began to see some shades and shapes. Hades always had people drink from the spring of forgetting so they would not miss their previous lives on earth. But Persephone started leading them to a special spring of memory so they could retain at least a memory of someone they loved. Because she remembered love, Persephone began to find the freedom to live in the cold, dark world.

Demeter missed her daughter terribly and refused to grow the crops needed to support the people of the earth. Eventually Zeus, Persephone's father and ruler of the gods, determined that Persephone would live part time in the underworld and part time on earth, so people would have crops to eat. She would live in both the dark, cold realm of death and in the light and warmth of life.

Persephone found a way to live in both the light and the dark. That was my challenge. Could I be like Persephone, the part-time Queen of Hades, finding a way to give color, life, spring, and summer to what promised to be a cold winter? Might I combine my fear and darkness with light and joy? I realized I must. Persephone's story had to become my story.

Over the following 18 months after I came to this realization, I tried to make sense of this contradiction: learning how to live in Hades and on earth, to bring sorrow and joy together, to die and live well at the same time. As Persephone did, I had to find a way across the river that was keeping me in despair. Making that transition is the subject of this chapter.

Drawing On My Cognitive Reserve

It was during my second session with my neuropsychologist, Dr. Schneiders, that he first brought up the concept of cognitive reserve (as I mentioned in chapter 2). He told me that given my education, my occupation, and my way of being in the world, my brain should show strong resistance to damage, and that would help me preserve the quality of my life. He went on to tell me of an Alzheimer's patient he had seen for 20 years whose cognitive reserve was strong.

Given that I still thought my darkness and misery were imminent, I was not so sure I wanted to live for 20 years. But to live the story of Persephone, I needed to return to that notion of cognitive reserve and learn what it meant. Harvard Health explains that cognitive reserve helps you be mentally agile and draw upon a lifetime of learning and thinking to identify more than one way of completing a task, a key to successfully coping with life's challenges.[1]

One of my favorite books on this disease is *A Tattoo on My Brain: A Neurologist's Personal Battle against Alzheimer's Disease* by Daniel Gibbs, a retired clinical neurologist who treated those with Alzheimer's and then found himself being the patient. Like me, Dr. Gibbs scored better on the cognitive tests than the imaging studies indicated he might. There was a discrepancy, so to speak, between the level of function indicated by his test scores and how he performed in daily life versus how the scans indicated he *should* be performing. Somehow he was outperforming expectations, which was attributed to cognitive reserve. Dr. Gibbs explains the theory of cognitive reserve this way:

> Another theory suggested that lifetime habits of study and stretching to learn, and other stimulating cognitive activity, contribute to the so-called cognitive reserve, a kind of brain bank of neural cells or networks that provided a backup, or created resilience, that might be keeping my cognitive functioning high despite the presence of brain atrophy and accumulations of plaques and tangles normally seen in mild to moderate Alzheimer's disease.[2]

Cognitive reserve is a theory, but more and more studies suggest that the brain can increase its resilience. Just as in some situations of stroke or other brain injury, a brain afflicted with Alzheimer's might create new pathways and find new circuits.

According to researchers, factors contributing to cognitive reserve include higher levels of education; professional occupation; and social, communal, and intellectual engagement. The more I learned about cognitive reserve, the more I appreciated how privileged I was. Not only do I have a PhD but I have also taught, written books, and worked at the highest levels of complex management. My jobs required me to be socially and intellectually engaged, and all my adult life I have been engaged in meaningful religious activities.

This is a real privilege, and I know the vast majority of people do not have the opportunity for this kind of education, occupation, and even intellectual engagement. But I don't want to minimize the fact that people without such education (people like my father) can be lifetime learners, can have intense friendships, and can participate in rich community life. The common denominator is curiosity, learning, and engagement.

Having all the education and intellectual engagement is helpful, but not necessary. Cognitive reserve can be created many ways. Everyone and anyone can build their reserve through reading, active learning, curiosity, travel, and doing things that stretch one's mind.

Strengthening cognitive reserve is like building stronger muscles. Yes, there are strengthening exercises you can do to build the muscles directly (which in this case translates to doing activities that cause your brain to stretch). But athletes and coaches will be the first to tell you that lifting weights alone does not make the muscles stronger; it requires diet, focus, sleep, and a host of other factors.

Stay healthy and learn—that is the key. For me to become Persephone, I had to stay healthy and learn new things. Learning is an opportunity for me (and for you!).

Contributions from My Inner Student and Educator

You may not have realized you were reading a book about the liberal arts, but I think this book is the most important act of a life and career dedicated to the liberal arts. The liberal arts is a tradition that dates back to the ancient Greeks. It was, until recently, the foundation of almost all undergraduate programs in the United States. The liberal arts are designed to prepare people—citizens—for a well-lived life. It assumes people can best serve themselves and their community when they learn to think critically, to cultivate a life of virtues and even excellence, and to appreciate all the different talents, perspectives, and work needed in our world. While I have tremendous respect for professional education like law and medicine and vocational education for so many critical trades, the liberal arts approach teaches one how to learn; it prepares one for a lifetime of learning.

Liberal arts is about gaining eyes to see the world in new ways, tools to live in the light, and skills to explore and build life forward.

My favorite story about education and a life worth living is the allegory of the cave in Plato's *Republic*. In this myth, Socrates describes certain people living as prisoners underground in a cave, chained by the neck and legs, facing the walls in darkness, a fire behind them providing only the dim shadows of life. The prisoners of the cave can only see the shadowy images of what people carry past the cave on a raised platform. When a prisoner is liberated, he is freed to see into the light. It causes pain and confusion.

From shadows, chains, and darkness, freedom is defined as seeing the light. Life, a life worth living, is made for seeing and living into the light. Knowledge is freedom to walk into the light and power to live fully.

For almost all my adult life—ages 28 to 68—I was an educator. Even when I held administrative positions at colleges and universities, I still saw my role as that of a learner and a teacher. Whether I was in the classroom, at a board meeting, around the table with faculty and staff, or on the road visiting alumni and parents, my job was to share information, cultivate discussion, and learn from others. Teaching was another role I thought I had lost—was taken away from me—the moment I retired.

Now as I work on this book, and after having just turned 71, I realize I am still a learner-teacher. I hope I have helped to share knowledge and insights that will empower those with Alzheimer's and their families. I have written this as an act of love for those who suffer from this disease and those who love them. I hope this work contributes to a community of Alzheimer's advocates who will let their voices be loud and their lives be filled with joy and meaning.

Beginning to Plan for the Future

While struggling to process the news, Fred and I had to make practical plans for our future. For Fred, it was a way of making sure I could be cared for in the best way. For me, it was largely wanting him to be situated as well as he could be for the dreaded journey he was about to take as my chief care partner. I am going to become a big burden, and I started to worry early on about how he would be supported through all this.

So, like Persephone in the winter months, we retreated to a dusky, dark, and cold Hades. We rewrote our wills and signed all the papers we could (especially me) about no extra life support. We talked to our financial advisors to make sure we were situated if I needed long-term care. Though I was constantly thankful for the ability to sign such papers and make such plans while I was fully cognizant, it felt and feels very dark and morbid to have conversations about planning for my demise. Signing my rights, my life, *myself* away. But it had to be done. And we are among the fortunate because our career paths have positioned us to navigate all of this with relatively comfortable retirement and other savings.

At that point, we were living in a large condo in downtown Denver that we had bought in order to entertain various groups as part of my role as chancellor at DU. On the 27th floor with large windows facing west, we enjoyed a panoramic view of the Rocky Mountains, and we could walk to some of the best restaurants in town. Fred and I began to discuss how the busyness and loudness of a large condo building in a downtown area was increasingly hard for me to deal with. Plus, it was more space than we needed now that our lives had become smaller. We loved being in the same building as my sister, Kathy, and her husband, Bob. The convenience of being able to see Kathy several times a week, to work out together or simply visit each other, was special. Fred and I weighed many options. We were especially concerned about what would happen when he couldn't care for me anymore. A sobering point.

We made the decision to move to a senior community that had independent living, assisted living, and memory care—thinking that we would then be prepared for any scenario. We selected a nice community and left downtown Denver for a beautiful new facility half an hour away.

The other residents, all at least fifteen years older than us, had all sorts of interests and talents. I joined the choir, attended the art groups, worked out in the fitness center, and went to various activities. We had to eat one meal a day from the kitchen, and though the food was good, the menu was limited. That got old very fast for both of us. We had jumped into that decision too early. Our own fear of the end drove us to a decision that didn't work for us. Though it was a lovely community, our lives had become too small too quickly. It didn't feel like we were living with joy or making the best use of the "good time" we still seemed to have left.

Luckily, we were renting. Deciding not to give up any more joy than we had to, we bought a home in a beautiful over-55 active-life-style community. The single home offered more space for me to paint, read, and write. We were closer to my son and daughter-in-law but still fairly close to my sister. I quickly made friends with great neighbors. I got a puppy (more about that later) and could walk him on all the trails through and around our community. And I could still enjoy my beloved mountain views. Fred did a great deal of research about in-home care and decided that, when the time came, we could do that for quite a while before needing to rethink our living situation. Our home is a great fit for us for now.

Carving a Path Out of the Underworld

The Persephone myth is interpreted in many ways, from an allegory for the four seasons to a story about the mother–daughter relationship. But for me it became a way of thinking about being in this underworld of knowing how I will die (the slow, long death of Alzheimer's) while also living with light and color. I still see the cold, dim shapes of how I will die, and yet I also have the freedom to surround myself with life, with color, with joy.

If you let just one voice break through the fog and haze of despair, let it be this one: the part of yourself that knows there's a battle to be fought—a battle worth fighting.

I have always found it helpful to have a narrative—a story or an allegory of sorts—to live through, to help me imagine my future. I find it a useful tool to help myself step back, see things more objectively, and remember that there are paths forward, even in the most rugged terrain. That's why I've adopted as my story or narrative the myth of Persephone, that resilient goddess who, consigned to the cold darkness of Hades, still returned to earth to live in the warmth of light and colors, even if only for a season or two at a time.

I hope you will come to the same realization that I did. That I couldn't—can't—just live in the underworld. I know some people remain in despair and distress, unable to imagine another path, giving in to the inevitable decline even before it arrives. The accompanying stress and depression, I think, hasten the progression of the disease and make life so very hard on one's loved ones.

Knowledge can take awhile to sink in, to be processed, to take hold.

Still, I felt a vague hope for a good life—for a while, maybe some years. I began to see into the light, even while darkness swirled around my ankles. I've managed to find a way to accept reality while soaking up as much life as I can. It's not easy, and it's not constant. But I write this book in part to help others see their situation afresh—just as Persephone began to see in new ways, even in an underworld she could not permanently escape. I, too, am working to find ways to spend time in the light, as I'll discuss in the next chapters.

Find Something to Inspire You

Because of my background, education, and a good friend's advice, I found inspiration in Greek myths. If Persephone can inspire you as well, that's great. But if not, find something that will. What story, what myth, what movie, what book will inspire you to move into the light, away from darkness? Perhaps a real or imagined rebel you've long admired? Or a beloved and admired friend who has somehow managed to keep living even after tragedy has struck?

6

What I've Learned about the Science of Alzheimer's Disease

AS SOMEONE WHO SOLVED complex problems for a living, I knew I had to have facts. While not a scientist or a neurologist, I decided to investigate Alzheimer's disease and dementia and do my best to understand what was going on with my brain so I could develop a degree of comfort and confidence in my choices about my lifestyle, treatments, and so on.

I was hoping to get insights to answer one of the most pressing questions I faced: Would research bring a fix, and what could I possibly do to help myself? An even better way to address my own flaming fears, I knew, would be to see if I could regain any semblance of control—doing anything at all that might make a difference.

My partner on this learning journey was and is Dr. Ann-Charlotte Granholm-Bentley (Lotta), a neurology researcher when I first met her. (She later became the first director of the Knoebel Institute for Healthy Aging at the University of Denver, as I'll discuss in a later chapter. Lotta was and continues to be incredibly helpful to me in understanding my diagnosis.) Lotta was already a friend before I received my diagnosis, and I knew I could trust her. So I revealed to her that the "complex neurological condition" referenced in my public statements was actually Alzheimer's (she had already assumed as much). I also asked her to explain what was happening in my brain.

Lotta, who speaks softly with a lovely Swedish lilt and a ready smile, came to my DU office with a notebook filled with pictures, studies, facts, language, and even some things I could *do*! I have kept in close touch with Lotta, who is definitely on my support team, and she allowed me to interview her for this book. Through her, I have learned that researchers and neurologists have many different opinions about what causes Alzheimer's, what the status of research for a cure really is, and even what can be done to help an Alzheimer's patient. With Lotta as my guide and interpreter, I continue to learn about Alzheimer's. Knowledge of the disease is ever expanding around how it can be mitigated by lifestyle interventions, and which frontiers of research seem closest to finding a cure. Allow me to share some of what I've learned that I hope you'll find helpful.

What Is Alzheimer's Disease?

Alzheimer's is a type of dementia, a general clinical term for a loss of memory, problem-solving abilities, language, and other brain functions that interfere with daily activities. Generally, dementia is the progressive loss of at least two cognitive abilities. It affects different individuals differently.

While most who suffer from dementia have short-term memory loss, they can also struggle with basic math and spatial-temporal disorientation (getting lost or forgetting the date), or experience paranoia and disturbing hallucinations. Some people will have trouble navigating social situations, as their ailing brain struggles to filter out noises and faces in the midst of commotion. This explains some of the changes I experienced that I didn't realize at first were symptoms of the disease, including, as I discussed in chapter 2, my growing reluctance to attend large social events, which had become more than I could bear because it had begun to feel as if every noise on earth was invading my skull.

Dementia has many faces and is a description used in many diseases and disorders of the brain. Here are the names of some of the conditions that I ran across in my research:

- Alzheimer's

- Lewy body dementia

- frontotemporal disorders

- chronic traumatic encephalopathy (CTE)

- Wilson's disease

- Huntington's disease

- Parkinson's disease

Any of these forms of dementia can lead to depression, and there's even a form of depression (pseudodementia) that mimics dementia.

Though Alzheimer's used to be thought of as an old person's disease, it can be diagnosed as early as one's forties or fifties. It is now thought that Alzheimer's disease pathology in the brain begins decades before any symptoms can be detected.

Scientists generally agree that the brain of someone with Alzheimer's has two types of cellular-level changes:

- **Amyloid plaques**—Amyloid is a naturally occurring protein in the brain. But in brains affected by Alzheimer's disease, the amyloid proteins form abnormal clumps between the nerve cells (neurons), which interrupt cell function.

- **Tau tangles**—Tau refers to a different kind of naturally occurring protein that helps transport nutrients and other molecules *inside* the nerve cells. In Alzheimer's disease, these tau proteins start sticking to each other, forming tangles, and they can no longer perform their primary function very well.

In short, both amyloid plaques and tau tangles are protein aggregations that lead to nerve cell loss and interfere with the way brain cells send and receive signals. As synapses (chemical or electric reactions that allow neurons to pass a signal) fail and neurons die, brain damage occurs.

To make this all worse, the cells within the brain that are responsible for immune responses—the microglia cells and astrocytes—react to the amyloid plaques just as they would an injury. Meaning the plaques stimulate inflammation, which further damages the brain. More and more research indicates the role of brain inflammation as contributing to the onset and progression of Alzheimer's. Inflammation can also be triggered or exacerbated by stress, disease, poor diet, lack of fitness, environmental factors such as pesticides, and food additives. And this explains why the refrain I heard from every neurologist, neuropsychologist, and researcher was: "Reduce the stress and you will live better and longer (most likely)."

NIH Definition of Alzheimer's Disease

For those of you who, like me, find comfort in knowing the science, here is the National Institutes of Health's description of Alzheimer's disease:[1]

> Alzheimer's is a progressive brain disorder that slowly destroys memory and thinking skills. Alzheimer's is characterized by the presence of two signature brain lesions: plaque deposits between nerve cells composed of fragments of the protein, amyloid beta (Aß), and neurofibrillary tangles (NFT) composed of aggregated tau proteins in the interior of cells.

Though the cellular changes associated with Alzheimer's are becoming better understood, scientists don't agree on what causes those changes nor how they can be prevented or reversed (cured). Researchers who focus on the amyloid plaques believe that reducing or dissolving these plaques will cure Alzheimer's. Those focused on the tau tangles believe the disease cannot be treated or cured until we find a way to untangle and eliminate them. (Dr. Granholm-Bentley says that the first group are referred to as beta amyloid "Baptists," and the second group are called "Taoists"—a bit of research humor. But the levity reflects the fact that despite strong convictions by both sets of researchers, there is no proof which theory is correct as of yet.)

In truth, it's likely there are multiple causes. Perhaps, as Dr. Granholm-Bentley argues, Alzheimer's is like a dystopian orchestra where different combinations of instruments perform different songs in different ways in different patients. Maybe Alzheimer's is a "family" of brain diseases, and there is not going to be just one cure.

Diagnosing Alzheimer's

Today, Alzheimer's can only be found and diagnosed after its effects have begun. Most often, patients seek a doctor's counsel after they notice symptoms ranging from forgetfulness and struggling with day-to-day activities to behavioral changes. Occasionally, as in my case, an observant physician notices early indicators and begins the testing process. My fervent hope is that a baseline memory test will become a standard part of annual physicals. Imagine how much earlier people could start to intervene in the progression of the disease if routine tests provided earlier warning.

In addition to memory tests, neurologists rely on either a lumbar puncture (spinal tap) or a PET scan of the brain to help diagnose Alzheimer's. Soon, biomarkers in the blood may be able to indicate at least the propensity, if not the actual presence, of the disease. For now, even the diagnosis of Alzheimer's is a guessing game, especially in the early stages. Many doctors will use the language of Mild Cognitive Impairment, waiting until the disease progresses to a moderate stage to give the diagnosis of Alzheimer's.

In fact, some experts say there is an inherent hesitance among physicians to give the diagnosis of Alzheimer's disease, perhaps due to the lack of effective treatment. This is similar to what happened with cancer diagnoses a few decades ago. In a time before there were widespread and effective treatments for many types of cancer, people's fear of the disease seemed to outweigh their desire to know what was going on because the knowledge didn't convey the power to do anything. However, just as with cancer treatments today, delaying the diagnosis of Alzheimer's prevents even the possibility of lifestyle interventions, treatment of symptoms, and (eventually, hopefully) a cure.

A National Health Challenge

According to the 2023 Alzheimer's Disease Facts and Figures, 6.7 million Americans live with this disease. Over 11 million Americans provide unpaid care. One in three seniors die with Alzheimer's—more than breast cancer and prostate cancer combined. In 2023, Alzheimer's and other dementias will cost the nation $345 billion. By 2050, these costs could rise to nearly $1 trillion.[2]

Some Encouraging Developments

Though I craved knowledge about Alzheimer's, the information alone didn't lead me out of Hades! Learning the medical descriptions and seeing pictures of sticky plaques accumulating in my brain brought me no peace. Seeing tau tangles choking my brain cells to death made me realize that the most precious part of my body—my essence—was degenerating, dying, soon to be filled with holes and empty spaces. Hades seemed even darker.

Because I had been a public figure in Denver who was now becoming known for my advocacy work with Alzheimer's, I was interviewed on Colorado Public Radio. Ryan Warner, the interviewer, told me he didn't think he would want to know if he had this disease, since there is no cure and nothing that can be done. Who would want to know about the diagnosis? Many echo that thought. I understand it. Many doctors don't even want to diagnose the disease, as there is no proven treatment for it. But, as scary as that knowledge is, there *are* some things to do, and those things helped me find the path to "living well," even in the face of the inevitable.

There are hopeful developments. Research for the treatment, prevention, and cure is exploding. We live in a time when the human brain is the great frontier of research. Much of this relates directly or indirectly to Alzheimer's. Monoclonal antibody (mAb) drugs are providing new avenues of treatment. MAb drugs are lab-made proteins designed to act like our natural antibodies (meaning they target sources of inflammation). Currently, mAbs that target the beta-amyloid proteins—those that form clumps between nerve cells—are especially promising. The drug Aduhelm (aducanumab) was approved in June 2021 by the FDA, albeit in the midst of some controversial findings and after a difficult clinical trial. A second drug, Leqembi (lecanemab), received traditional FDA approval on July 6, 2023. To be specific, this drug received accelerated approval in January 2023, but until July 2023, Medicare had blocked access to both drugs (Aduhelm and Leqembi) in its coverage policies. As of this writing, a third mAb drug, donanemab, is on the horizon for FDA approval sometime soon. Even with the support of Medicare, these drugs are costly and only effective for some people. But the approval of these mAb drugs represents a historic breakthrough: treatment is on the horizon.

Other drug-based treatments are also being investigated. I hope that until this disease is cured, there will continue to be new research programs developed to reduce and prevent Alzheimer's. Given the aging population of baby boomers, there is incredible incentive—financial and otherwise—to find effective treatments or cures. As we continue to learn more about Alzheimer's, it will be treated more like cancer, heart disease, and so many other treatable diseases. More effective treatments might also mean that doctors will hesitate less to offer a diagnosis—and fewer patients will opt to live in denial, under the false premise that there is nothing they can do about it anyway. But for now, the research hasn't found any way to stop, let alone reverse, the progress or prevent the disease through pharmacological treatment, a vaccine, or preventive pill. But the research is promising, and I see this as a sign of great hope.

But hope of future progress wasn't going to get me across the bridge from the darkness of Hades into the light of earth. That transition began with my research on lifestyle intervention and its relation to cognitive reserve. This research does not provide a cure—though we all wish it were that straightforward. But I learned from Dr. Granholm-Bentley and others that I might be in a position to preserve the quality of my life and prolong the "good years" of living with Alzheimer's before the final stages of not knowing, not remembering, and being totally dependent took over. Not a cure, but still potentially a merciful gift.

Moving Forward with Imperfect Knowledge

My parents used to say of me, "she is too busy to sit." Though I now move more slowly and sleep 12 hours a day, for most of my life I never sat still unless I had a good book to keep my mind occupied. I used to imagine my brain as a giant Pac-Man, gobbling up all the bits of knowledge and information I could. And even though my brain is developing tangles, plaques, and who knows what else, I still am restless to take the next step.

My layperson's summary about the science of Alzheimer's is that we don't know the cause or causes of the disease. Heck, we can't even know definitively if one has the disease until a patient dies and an autopsy is performed. There are no cures yet, though we know that keeping inflammation down helps. And we know, without any doubt, this disease is both real and devastating. This is the paradox that those of us with Alzheimer's live with: this disease is both a mystery and an all-consuming reality. It's a bit like Persephone's dual citizenship in Hades and on earth.

I admit that learning about tau and tangles, plaque and amyloids was a bit challenging and perhaps not relevant for everyone. As my knowledge grew and I began to understand more and more what was happening inside my brain, I was flabbergasted to find there is no known cause. Indeed, there may be no one cause. I am reminded of Lotta's "dystopian orchestra" concept, unique to every person who suffers from this disease. Sometimes I can picture what is going on in my brain as a bunch of screeching instruments playing off-key without harmony or melody.

That said, as I read carefully through scientific reports about research regarding treatment, I saw some hope in the promising pharmacological treatments being developed, and more and more treatments being tested. The more I read and talked and thought about the implications of all this new information, the less I felt like I was destined to drift quickly into oblivion. I began to believe that we are on the cusp of some effective medical treatments. I doubt there will be one magic pill for everyone. And even with treatment, lifestyle interventions will still be needed, but that is no different than any other chronic condition such as living with heart disease.

I still dread my Hades—this particular kind of death sentence where I will lose my mind, my memories, myself, likely all before my body begins to fail. I remained scared of getting lost, gazing out the window for hours, being led around by others. But—importantly—I was not (and am not) there yet.

Armed with so much new knowledge, I had a choice to make: I could descend quietly into Hades, wallow in the lack of a cure, and despair at whether any steps I could take would help prolong the quality of my life. Or I could spend my time creating flowers on earth. I chose to fight. And I found new avenues for stretching my brain through art, creativity, and spirituality, which have brought even more light into my life, as I'll discuss in the next chapters.

7

"You Need to Learn to Paint"

"Every child is an artist; the problem is staying an artist when you grow up."

—ATTRIBUTED TO PABLO PICASSO

I DON'T WANT TO FORGET FRANCES. *I met Frances when I was at Emory. She became the VP for student affairs and, several years after she arrived, I became provost and VP for academic affairs. We were the first women vice presidents in the history of this very southern and rather conservative university.*

Frances is a big personality, full of energy, insight, and creativity. Her very laugh makes my heart smile. She is compassionate beyond words. How many homeless and otherwise struggling students did she support out of her own purse? I know there were many. We rocked the president's staff a bit, who were all men who didn't quite expect our smarts and our humor to be at the decision-making table every day. Franny and I became fast and deep friends, laughing through victories and crying through the inevitable failures and losses in life. After my diagnosis, Frances decided she would teach me to paint. And painting is one of the best gifts anyone has ever given me.

But I will forget Franny's face, her stately presence, that gorgeous laugh. I will forget, too, the gift she gave me in teaching me how to load paint on my brush, how to create depth by different values, and how to layer colors.

My friend Frances Lucas called me during the time when Fred and I were starting to make decisions about the next steps for my life and death with Alzheimer's. She informed me that I needed to learn to paint, as that would help my brain by forcing it to flex and make new connections. Frances had been painting for some years and had learned how good painting is for the soul and for getting your brain to stretch in new ways.

Spoiler alert! I did eventually learn to paint. It wasn't an easy or quick path, though I will tell you up front that the struggles were well worth it. The first steps were hardest because I had to overcome a lifetime of belief that I had no artistic skills.

Art as a Spectator Sport

I have loved art most of my life, but until recently had enjoyed it as a spectator not as a participant.

I grew up in a home without art on the walls. We had no art books on the coffee table. The first time I saw "art" was in the third grade at Jessie Clark Elementary. We went on a field trip to the Wichita Museum of Art. What struck me viscerally was the medieval painting of a crucified Jesus being carried off the cross. It wasn't that it was about Jesus, for I had little biblical or theological knowledge at that age. There was something about the cerulean blue sky, the amber red in the robes, and the slow, haunting movement of the men. Even as an eight-year-old who had never really seen art before, the draping of the clothing absorbed me. I just wanted to stand there and look at it forever. The teacher had to pull me by the arm to make sure I kept up with the class.

Years later, I was in a philosophy class in college and turned the page of a chapter on abstraction and saw a brilliant orange and blue Mark Rothko painting on the left-hand side of the page. "What in the world?" I thought. On the thin page of this cheap paperback book, whose name I've long forgotten, this picture shimmered. I don't remember any of the words in that chapter or even what I learned in that class, but I vividly recall the sheer joy I felt in staring at the picture of this painting.

For years, I lugged that philosophy book with me through all my moves so I could keep looking at that picture. Like the painting I saw in third grade, this painting is burned into my memory and soul. (As with everything else I discuss in this book, I know that Alzheimer's will steal that memory from me, but until then I will remember that moment of first seeing the Rothko painting. Thinking of it reignites feelings of joy, peace, and groundedness.)

But while I appreciated the talent of others, I firmly believed I had no such talent myself. I had never so much as picked up a paintbrush, so Frances's order that I learn to paint seemed impossible to me

I (Reluctantly) Learn to Paint

Frances announced (as only she could) that my exploration of painting would begin by taking a trip to Crested Butte, Colorado. We would stay in a house her brother owned, and I could invite two friends. I love Frances, and I knew there was no way to decline this invitation. Also, Crested Butte is one of my favorite places to hike.

Without much thought, I brushed aside the invitation to paint, and did so without regret or remorse. I figured I would just have to give Frances some painting companions. I had to pick two friends who would also like to hike, who would be fun, who would not make a big deal about my diagnosis—and who might be willing to paint with Frances while I went hiking or read or made myself useful by cooking meals. I was starting to realize that I had the freedom to do what I needed to do for myself, even with my friends!

I ended up inviting my sister, Kathy, who, according to my mother, was the real artist in the family. (In my mother's view, I most definitely was not an artist.) I also invited Serene Jones, a friend of mine who is president of Union Theological Seminary in New York City. I never got to see enough of Serene, so this would be a great opportunity—especially because I knew Serene was on sabbatical and therefore might actually have the time. I didn't know if Serene painted, but I imagined she would at least dabble. She is incredibly creative in all that she does. And I knew she loved to hike. Like me, she also loved to cook. So if nothing else, she could go hiking and do the cooking with me.

Kathy and Serene agreed, each of them excited. My goal was accomplished: we would have fun, and Frances would have companions for her painting.

We arrived on a beautiful late August day in 2019, surrounded by the majestic Rockies. Crested Butte is the wildflower capital of Colorado, and all around us the landscape was in bloom. We drove to a high pass and let the wind try to blow us off the mountains. When we first got to the house, we ate, we drank, we laughed.

Then the moment arrived: "Ladies, let's get painting!" Frances boomed out. Kathy and Serene eagerly took their places at the table. I casually said that I was going to read while they were painting, and then

I would cook dinner for everyone. Instantaneously, and all together, Frances, Kathy, and Serene objected—it felt like a coup. Even my sister, who knows how deeply sensitive I am to having to do things I will not be good at, insisted that I paint with them. "It doesn't matter what you paint," "It's all just for fun," and so on. Ugh!

I don't know that I had ever really thrown a tantrum in my life until that moment. I had an absolute fit. I was angry, embarrassed, and a bit out of control. I sat and watched while Frances painted a beautiful landscape. Kathy selected a picture of a Georgia O'Keeffe painting and did a rendition that Georgia would have approved. Serene did another O'Keeffe and even glued shells and other things to the ox skull she painted. Oh my! They were painting effortlessly and giggling constantly. Kathy hadn't painted since she was in high school, and Serene had never painted. As I watched their flair and their fun, my fear and my resistance skyrocketed.

What I didn't realize until that moment was that Frances's determination was even stronger than my resistance. She would not be deterred. Frances is tall, with a strong, powerful physical presence. From Mississippi, she has a strong southern twang and a commanding voice. She can make a room laugh, cry, or go completely quiet with her facial expressions and tone of voice.

She said, "Honey child, I am going to sit here with you, and we are going to paint that pretty flower together. Don't you worry: you will make a beautiful flower." I tried to paint a sunflower in a red pot. The pot was misshapen, the sunflowers uneven, with flat yellow splotches.

I became an unholy mess. Why didn't they just let me be? Could they not see that I was an utter failure at this? Why should I even try? Why did they insist on humiliating me? Just let dementia kill me now!

Gently (if infuriatingly, at first), Frances would suggest ideas to me. She would take the paintbrush and frequently murmur, "Hmmm" as she used it to help me transform my little sunflower. She put a lot more paint on the canvas and varied the colors in the flowers and in the pot. She showed me where to put highlights and add a background. At the end of two days of work, I had created a six-by-six-inch lonely sunflower on an irregular, red-striped background.

Then Frances wanted us to paint another picture. I really didn't want to but also didn't want to hurt her feelings after she had given me so much help, and I certainly didn't want to dampen the mood of everyone else, especially after my initial outburst. Kathy, Serene, and Fran were having a great time: listening to music, dancing around, painting with abandon. I felt like a heavy stone trying to be a graceful butterfly. But, always a good girl and really loving my friends, I limped along. Frances and I painted a small mountain landscape together. Now, when I say we painted *together*, I really mean that I would smash some paint on the canvas, and Frances would use her deft touch to fix it into something recognizable.

I don't remember if I enjoyed doing this second painting, but I discovered I liked the smell and the feeling of the paint. I loved all the colors, and somehow the creativity involved lured me more and more into feelings of hope and joy and peace. Much to my surprise, painting created a good kind of forgetting where I could leave behind all the worries and stresses of everyday life. As one friend, Susan Sharpe, later told me, painting is like resting in the heart of God.

I began to realize painting, at least for me, didn't have to be about producing good art; it could be about enjoying the process of moving into the world of light, of colors, of joy, of peace, and of hope. (It's almost as though Frances knew from the beginning not only that painting would be good for me, but also that I could lose myself in the pure joy of it.)

Painting Grabs Hold

When we returned from our painting trip to Crested Butte—where I learned against my will that I could produce something at least better than the work of a young child—Kathy and I decided to keep painting. We had talked off and on over the years, noncommittally, that painting or drawing or pottery might be something we could do when we were both retired.

During the fall of 2019, we began playing with art in the most basic way. We bought some inexpensive acrylic paints and canvases, got easels (that's what made us feel like real painters), and started identifying videos with simple lessons we could follow. At that point, I was fortunate to have a large space to dedicate to painting. I found a woman who called herself The Art Sherpa,[1] who could make even the most inexperienced painter feel comfortable. The Art Sherpa, with pink and purple hair and plenty of tattoos, gives detailed instructions and shares lots of encouraging and fun ideas, but it was hard work for me.

My first painting under The Art Sherpa's virtual tutelage was from her video *Easy Girl Acrylic Painting*. The video, labeled as entry level, runs about one hour. Contrary to what the title implied, for me there was nothing easy about it! I worked and worked on it. It took me *weeks* to paint this simple girl, really a caricature of a girl. I painted and repainted the hair, the eyes, the mouth, and the contours of the body. Fortunately, acrylic paint is forgiving because you can just white out your mistakes and paint over them. It was hard, but I also found it fun—so I kept going. I was pleased with the painting, even though it was just a start. You can see the result of my efforts in Figure 7.1.

FIGURE 7.1:
MY "EASY GIRL" PAINTING

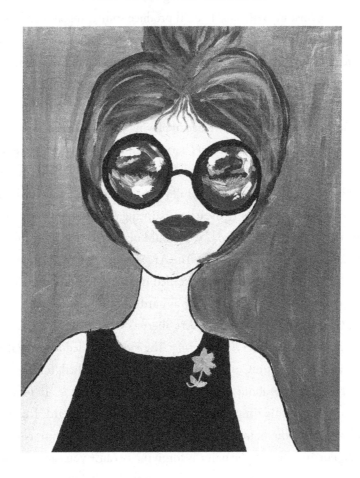

My sister and I also followed videos by Emma Petitt, who paints deliberately misshapen women using the vibrant colors of turquoise, orange, lime green, and burnt red. Some friends with Alzheimer's tell me they see colors more vividly as the disease progresses, and I have experienced a similar phenomenon. Kathy and I would splash Petitt's wild colors on the canvas, spray the wet paint with water, and watch the colors bleed together. Then we would sketch out a woman with huge hands, or oversized thighs, and always wild, wild hair. This didn't take precision. It only required that you suspend what a woman "ought" to look like. I called mine my Wacky Ladies, displayed them on top of my kitchen cabinets, and smiled as my husband raised his eyebrows and kept his comments to himself. I also experimented with other subjects after watching Emma's videos, which led to the curious dog (Figure 7.2), which I did in black-and-white shades, and a full-color red-haired woman (Figure 7.3), whose coloring you'll have to take for granted.

FIGURE 7.2
CURIOUS DOG

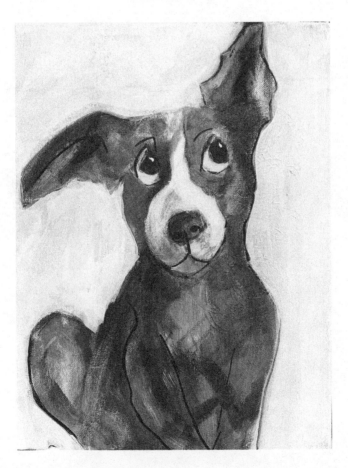

FIGURE 7.3
RED-HAIRED WOMAN

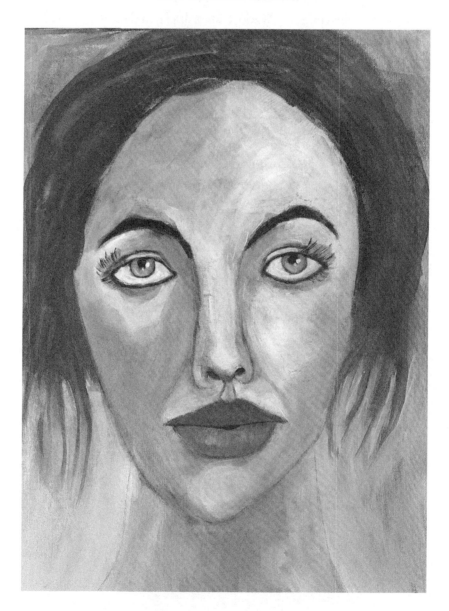

Discovering Freedom
When Outcome Doesn't Matter

The early stage of learning to paint was perhaps the first time in my life when the outcome of what I was doing didn't matter. There was no tenure committee or board of trustees to answer to, no group of faculty waiting to weigh in on my results. I enjoyed the process of painting, and I liked learning how to do it. I don't know that I realized it at the time, but painting stretched my brain in new ways, and new learning felt like a small victory over my diagnosis. The practice of painting, I quickly discovered, pulled me into itself. Time slowed down, my mind calmed, the colors swept over me, and the canvas welcomed me. Nothing else mattered when I had a brush or palette knife in my hand.

Upping Our Artistic Skills

Later that fall, Kathy suggested we up our game and take a class at the Student Art League of Denver during its winter session. We decided (probably due to my timidity) to take a course titled "Drawing for Those Who Think They Can't." The sessions were held in a cold, cavernous room in an old brick school building. At the opening session, I sat in the back. I was nervous to be a student again, sure that I would fail utterly (and knowing I hate to fail). I still believed in the myth that one had to have natural artistic talent in order to draw or paint. How could I begin to think I could paint when even my handwriting is nearly illegible?

In our first class, the teacher had us take a piece of paper, divide it into four squares, and do simple pencil drawings of our face, a cup, a vase, and a flower, each in its own quarter of the paper. Then we had to share them. How embarrassing! Mine were like a four-year-old's drawings. As I looked around, though, I noticed that some others had similar drawings, and that helped ease the humiliation.

The classes progressed. We learned to draw a cup, a still life, and a chair. We tried charcoal and pastels. We learned about values and negative spaces. Though I didn't find drawing to be as playful as painting, I experienced the pleasures of curiosity and learning. Yet again, I noticed I could feel my brain stretching in new ways. The practice of drawing was creating a new way of seeing and being. Every time I tried a new lesson, I felt my soul expanding and quieting at the same time. This was not at all what I had expected.

Near the end of the course, we had to draw another self-portrait, this time while looking in a mirror. I labored and labored. I had never seen my face so clearly or objectively. The picture I drew was a thousand times better than the one I had sketched on day one, and it definitely looked like me in a fairly realistic way (see Figure 7.4). I began to question my fundamental belief that I couldn't draw.

Have You Been Told You Can't Draw?

So many times when I talk about painting, I hear the comment, "I can't draw, I have no talent." But what if talent can be learned? What if we all have the potential to draw or sing or create and we just haven't developed it? Heck, even if some of us are innately "bad" at drawing, couldn't there still be value in learning how to unlock our inner creativity and maybe improve our skills?

FIGURE 7.4

MY FIRST AND LAST SELF-PORTRAITS FROM
THE STUDENT ART LEAGUE CLASS

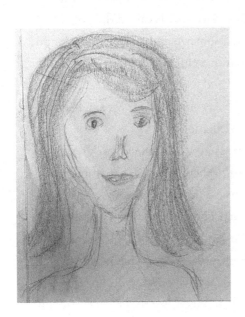 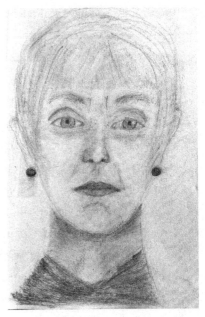

The first self-portrait I ever drew (left side) and the last self-portrait from my first class at the Student Art League of Denver. The class was specifically for people who think they can't draw, which I certainly was at the time. By the end of the class, I began to think (hope?) I had been wrong!

One recent Christmas, I gave a dear friend, Joyce, a small and simple painting of an angel that I had made. Like most of us when we receive a handmade gift in this world of cheaply manufactured goods, she was touched. This simple angel had no face and was set against a plain magenta background. And yet she raved about my talent. Joyce said she wished she could paint or draw, but she had no talent. I countered with all I had learned about the latent talents within us—lessons no one taught her (or me, until this point!). I argued that perhaps art teachers in grade school had convinced her she couldn't draw or paint. "Oh, no," Joyce said. "You have real talent." I replied that I really didn't, but I had learned to draw, paint, and see in a somewhat artistic way. Back and forth we went. Finally, I pointed out that children draw, paint, and sing and dance before they learn to read and write. "Oh," she said, "you are right; we do color before we read." Argument won! We laughed and went on with our festive evening celebration over a glass of wine.

Ever since, I have become attuned to watching young children enjoy their creativity. My gorgeous great-nephew Kairos Cole visited us in Denver when he was just 18 months old (this was several years after my diagnosis). This red-headed, blue-eyed, fair-skinned child with his happy temperament had already "painted" in his day care. I gave him some very big markers (ones that wash off easily) and a large tablet, and he happily stood at his father's knee and made colorful marks on the paper for a long time. Maybe I was seeing too much, but the colors worked in great combinations, and he made all sorts of different shapes with his bright, bold colors. The little fellow was practicing art, his right brain fully unleashed—and too young to be inhibited by self-doubt. Kairos knew quite a few words at that time but was not yet speaking complete sentences. As I had mentioned to Joyce, we color before we speak.

The capacity for this practice of painting and drawing and coloring (or any of the creative arts) is apparent in young children. It is also present throughout our lives, including among those who have Alzheimer's. We just need to learn, to pick up the crayons or the pencil or paint, get some cheap paper so we don't worry about the "cost" of mistakes, and begin. We also need to shed our inner monologue about whether we're "good enough" and just keep learning by coloring or painting—if it gives us joy.

Where Is Your Creative Spark?

I got into painting and drawing because my friend Frances was an angel who guided me . . . across the bridge between Hades and earth, from darkness into color and light. I began to glimpse, through the fog of my fear, that maybe while I lived, while I still had my wits about me, I could enjoy life. Maybe there was a chance I could focus on the quality of my life, if not the quantity of my remaining years.

Even with that glimpse of possibility and hope, I had to accept that the feelings of fear, depression, and sadness would bubble up often. They still do. I live in the light and warmth, surrounded by colors. I experience spring and summer. But the shadow of fall and darkness of winter visit me on occasion.

For me, the practice of creativity is through painting. But painting and art are not the only ways to tap into creativity. Music is a well-documented form of creative practice for those with Alzheimer's. Music often summons memories, even among those in advanced stages of the disease. Fred, my husband, is a retired pastor and used to visit congregants weekly in nursing homes. Many of the residents could no longer communicate, but they could join him in the hymns of their youth. Music memory, evidently, is one of the deepest memories in our brain.

Cooking a meal can be another form of creativity. In Virginia Woolf's novel *Mrs. Dalloway*, producing dinner parties was an art. In making a meal, you have to imagine the menu, find the recipes, organize the ingredients, and cook the food with care. One is surrounded by the colors, the smells, the textures, the sounds of water running, oil snapping in the pan. And then you set the table, perhaps with flowers and special plates. You seat your invited guests carefully, hoping for the best conversation over the feast.

Gardening is another beautiful practice of creativity. My grandmother, once a master gardener, lost many of her cognitive capacities, but she continued to visit her overgrown garden and feel the petals of her roses. The list of creative practices is almost endless: flower arranging, woodworking, car restoration, photography, cooking, and so on all calm the soul, connect the brain and body, stretch the mind, and allow one to see and be in new and expanded ways.

I love that all these creative practices invoke beauty. There are many different ways to be a Persephone and live in light and color, to be fed and feed others, and to experience beauty. Often as I paint, I imagine that my time with Alzheimer's has allowed me access to the beauty of the universe in a way I never before took the time to see. I believe that since my brain began changing, I have begun using more of its capacity even as some parts are being lost. Just what was going on is what I'll discuss in the next chapter.

What Will You Have the Courage to Try?

The biggest barrier to discovering my artistic side was my fear of failure. As I've mentioned, I had a lifelong pattern of not wanting to start things I was sure I would fail at. Big surprise—my fear had kept me from something that ended up fulfilling me in ways I couldn't anticipate. So my challenge for you is to think of a creative activity that fills you with fear, then try it. Don't worry about the outcome: the painting, the meal, the garden, what you look like on a dance floor. Focus on finding joy in the process.

8

Exploring the Right Side of My Brain

THE COURSE MY SISTER AND I TOOK at the Student Art League was based on a classic book called *Drawing on the Right Side of the Brain* by Betty Edwards. It was first published in 1979, but what most consider to be the "definitive" edition was released in 2012. This book is like the Bible for generations of students learning to draw. This magical book not only explains drawing and provides exercises, but it also teaches how drawing and painting can create new neural pathways or connections in the brain. In this chapter, I'll talk more about what I've learned about the left versus right brain metaphor and how it can help us think differently about what our brains are capable of.

Left versus Right Brain

Relying on the science available to her in the '70s, Edwards talks about the right side versus the left side of the brain. Today, scientists don't think there is a clear left/right brain duality. Rather, practices such as art and music draw upon various parts of the brain. Still, the left brain/right brain concept is an incredibly useful metaphor to talk about how art (and other creative activities) engages the brain through our physical activity in nonlinear, nonquantitative fashions. So I will continue to use the left/right brain terminology throughout this chapter.

In the metaphor of left/right brain, the left brain represents activities that require logical, systematic thinking, such as math, language, and speech, and more generally, thought, objectivity, and rationality. The right brain represents that which is intuitive, perceptive, imaginative, and subjective. As Edwards says, "You are probably familiar with the following ideas embedded in our languages and cultures. The main divisions are between thinking and feeling, intellect and intuition, and objective analysis and subjective insight."[1]

Edwards introduces the notion that objectivity and intuition are two distinct ways of knowing. In my career, I relied upon both: I would start objectively analyzing a problem or a possibility, weigh all the different pros and cons, dream of new approaches, consider how others would likely respond to solutions, and eventually figure out what my gut (intuition) was telling me. The best solutions came about when both my head and my heart were aligned, which I guess predestined me to easily believe that utilizing both left and right brain functions in our brains is the best way to increase cognitive reserve. I also thought back to the art that had impressed me in my youth and realized that though I didn't have the language of right brain/left brain at that point, those paintings had spoken directly to the right side of my brain.

In her book, Edwards takes readers through various exercises that turn off the left side of the brain so that the right side can express itself. The exercises are fascinating: attempting to copy a sketch that is upside down so you can't analyze it, drawing your hand without looking at it, and drawing a still life by only looking at the spaces in between the shapes and forms (negative space). As my teacher walked us through these and other exercises, I began to know and to see differently. And, amazingly, my drawing matured. They no longer looked like they came from a child with little coordination in her fingers!

The Loss of Right-Brain Education

In recent decades in the United States, a push for STEM (science, technology, engineering, and math) has coincided with a devaluing of holistic or liberal approaches. In other words, the right side of the brain has become less and less valued. Schoolchildren used to learn not only reading, writing, and arithmetic but also art and music. Now, given the cost of education and public perception of what subjects carry the most benefit for future careers, the least-valued subjects often get eliminated. Many children never have the opportunity to learn how to draw or sing, nor how to express feelings through a creative process. If they do not learn there are these two ways of knowing (or seeing) the world, they can't appreciate that essentially holistic way of bringing together the objective and the subjective, the rational and the intuitive, the heart and the head.

Life Imposes a Left-Brain Focus

While by nature I am predisposed to appreciate both right- and left-side thinking, for much of my adult life the requirements of my career and family imposed a need for left-brain function. This became true as soon as I entered graduate school at the University of Chicago Divinity School—which we students referred to as marine training for scholars. At that point, and ever since (until my diagnosis), left-brain thinking almost exclusively took over my life.

I was, after all, a working mother at that point, which requires a lot of executive management skills as well as the need to multitask and prioritize. I vividly remember the winter of 1983, which, until recently, had the coldest recorded day in Chicago's history with a wind chill of 32 degrees below zero. My days had been following a standard routine:

I got up at four o'clock to try to squeeze in two hours of work on my papers despite the frigid temperatures in my study. My husband and I would waken our son, make him some French toast or something else for breakfast, and then my husband, Mark, would leave for his church. I would bundle Nate up with multiple coats, surround him with blankets on his round red rubber sled, drag him to school, then return home so I could get my car and drive to the university campus. (This routine was broken once during 1983's Great Blizzard. My car would not start, so I walked with frozen feet to the divinity school. I had a floor-length canvas beige L.L. Bean coat that was, without a doubt, the world's ugliest garment. I covered my face with a thick gray wool ski mask that had holes for my eyes and topped off the ensemble with a very warm and cheap brown faux fur hat.)

At that time, I worked at an academic magazine, *The Journal of Religion*, in the basement of the divinity school building, where the radiators always put off intense heat. I was either freezing or sweating all day long. For lunch, I would gobble down the same lunch I always packed for my son: a peanut butter and jelly sandwich, though I added a Snickers bar and a cup of hot tea to complete my meal.

Like always when my husband, son, and I got home, I'd fix my son a snack, and he would play while I prepared dinner. After supper, we played some more until his bedtime, after which I was back down to the freezing cold basement study of our townhouse parsonage to work until midnight. That was a pretty standard day at that phase in my life. Having routines was the key to getting as much done every day as I could.

But even during this intensely left-brain period, there were two exceptions to my high-pressured routine where right-brain activity was required. The first had to do with playing with my son. On some weekends, while Mark attended to his parish duties, Nate and I would invent new worlds. We turned a storage unit into the *Millennium Falcon* and conquered the cosmos. On other weekends, Nate's many stuffed animals (each with its own name) were allowed to take over the house. The animals were the most amazingly accomplished creatures— they fought wars, slayed dragons, created churches, taught schools, and traveled to the four corners of the world. I loved those times, when my left brain turned off and my right was fully activated.

The other exception to my routine was visiting the Art Institute of Chicago, which was free on Thursdays. Occasionally, I would go off to the Art Institute, sometimes alone and sometimes with my husband. My favorite place was in front of the vivid Marc Chagall windows. The powerfully deep blues with splashes of reds, greens, and yellows comforted me, and the whimsical nature of his animals and people turned my right brain fully on. Even then, in the midst of all my busyness and considerable pressure from my graduate studies, art brought me peace, inspiration, and joy. As I became more able to afford the admission fee, trips to museums and art fairs became more frequent, and I began to read about artists. I purchased prints of Van Gogh paintings, and my husband and I bought several pieces of inexpensive abstract art. We had art on our walls! How in the world did these artists conceive of these creations, let alone bring them into being?

What I now realize is that my left brain was so fully engaged by graduate school and all my other activities that my own imagination was becoming more and more limited. Or at least, it was my left-brain functions that I told myself were critical throughout my professional life.

In retrospect, I realize I often had to rely on a creative spark to find solutions in my administrative jobs, just as I had built fortresses and jungles when playing with Nate when he was a child. For example, one trick I had learned as an administrator was to take intractable problems and reframe them into creative possibilities. When I arrived at Swarthmore College, one such problem was a 10-year-long battle to build an inn and restaurant next to the bucolic campus, situated in the suburbs of Philadelphia. There was no nearby hotel to host visitors, including parents and families coming to tour campus. There were limited dining options within walking distance. To make it all even more difficult in the academic community of Swarthmore, the few snack shops in town couldn't serve alcohol to even those over 21 because long ago the Quakers who had founded the college and town of Swarthmore had made it a dry community. It became apparent after I listened to faculty, staff, students, alumni, and others that we needed an inn. Unfortunately, many believed that the town of Swarthmore would be hurt and that residents would likely be opposed. After listening, I knew I had to reframe this issue so that others could see it as a win-win for all. Very carefully, I and some of the senior team began to talk to the leaders and residents of the town. We crafted plans so that the local community could benefit from the inn. We fixed a major traffic problem for them in our plans and ensured that our restaurant, bar (the first ever in this heretofore dry town), and bookstore would be of value to the broader community. After some time and consideration, the Swarthmore Inn became a beautiful hotel and restaurant for bringing the college and the community together.

Yet somehow the demands of the life of a senior educational administrator had made me discount my creative talents. It wasn't until I began painting that I realized how much of my self-identity was tied to my left-brain talents—and it was time I readjusted that image to include my right-brain creativity. It was time to continue my artistic journey.

Continuing the Path of Artistic Discovery

After my diagnosis, the need to further explore my right-brain functions has gained a new prominence in my life. And not just for the thrill of being creative. I found that picking up my brushes and painting almost always created a stillness in me and stretched my mind. So I continued with more videos, more dabbling, and found books to read and study. I took a few lessons with a local teacher, but before we could really get launched with our lessons, COVID ended our in-person sessions.

Fortunately, before we had to abruptly end our in-person lessons, the teacher told me of a book called *Learn to Paint in Acrylics with 50 Small Paintings: Pick Up the Skills, Put on the Paint, Hang Up Your Art* by Mark Daniel Nelson. When COVID narrowed our lives in so many ways, that book became my project—and a source of expanding my own mind and world. Nelson breaks down each lesson into four or five simple steps with pictures accompanied by excellent interpretations of the steps. Each lesson illustrates a basic point: color mixing, glazing, values, perceptions, and so on. These were all new words to me.

In lesson 10, on mixing tints and shades, I painted a gorgeous red poppy. (At that point, I had been painting for eight months and had never said "gorgeous" about anything I had painted.) Better yet, in lesson 35, I painted a transparent blue balloon dog. I still get comments on that dog!

Months later, during a lull between COVID outbreaks, my good friend Tom asked if he could buy a picture I had painted of the Great Smoky Mountains. I was tickled and of course gave it to him as a gift.

There were also many failures. My painting of a field and pasture looked like a green-and-yellow blob with an off-centered red square (supposedly a barn). I was so excited to paint a sunflower on my own (I am, after all, from the Sunflower State of Kansas), but I could not get the center of the flower proportionate to the petals, so at best it was an orange circle with brown dots and a yellow fringe.

Sometimes I would be discouraged with my lack of talent, and sometimes I feared that my brain was so diseased that attempting to learn something new was pointless. Most of the time, though, I was grateful for the ability to create. I was enchanted with the practice: the being and doing, the letting go while doing the work of creating. I had to keep reminding myself that the product didn't matter and the failures didn't count. The successes, which I had once in a while, were much more fun, but they didn't really count either. What mattered was the peace I felt in painting, the new skills I was acquiring, the joy it all gave me. And the way it helped my brain feel alive.

The Birth of a Portrait Artist

I loved my practice of art, but I didn't want to just repeat my wacky ladies or my amateur landscapes forever and ever. I went web surfing again, looking for ways to enhance my practice of art, stretch my mind with new skills, and bring peace to my soul. I must have looked at and rejected a hundred websites. Many were similar to what I was already doing; many just demanded too much money, paint, and expertise.

I kept thinking about art as capturing the image of people. I love the work of Alex Katz, whose bold paintings are so wonderful at capturing the living vibrancy of the people he paints. I began to wonder if I could master enough technique to paint some of my family members and friends. I had a vision of me in the later stages of my disease, surrounded by my paintings of those I loved. I could write out stories of each person that my loved ones could read to me. What a comforting, if daunting, thought: to paint my friends and family members!

One day, I found a blog called *Realistic Acrylic Portrait School*. I almost moved on to another site. I pride myself on being eclectic in all my tastes, but those Dutch masters and their realistic paintings never commanded my attention. But something drew me to the website. Matt Philleo is an artist and teacher who maintains the blog. I looked at his art and the offerings in his school.

Matt was offering a challenge where he posted videos of the process of painting a picture and invited followers to watch the videos and attempt the same painting. That spring the challenge was drawing Maka, a beautiful African American bride. I decided I'd at least try it. Matt paints in the style of the old Renaissance masters, using lots and lots of layers. He has updated this process using matte medium and acrylic paint. In order to speed up the process of drawing the sketch, you first draw a grid on your canvas and then sketch, inch by square inch. Then you start your many, many layers. Once you join the school, you have access to a weekly online session with other students to share feedback on their work—all guided by Matt.

I can't say I felt pure joy in this process, but there was something about the slow, meditative process of creating these layers. Who knew the delicate dance of the layers of these colors. And I had no idea that an eyelid off by an eighth inch would make a painting look so different! Matt was one of the best teachers I have ever had: encouraging, patient, technical, challenging, loving.

In January 2021 I jumped all in—not knowing if I would drown or swim—and signed up for weekly sessions. Matt is a devoted and thoughtful Christian whose practice of art is equally sensitive to the Creator and to human limits, with our strange combination of talents and trials. I would send what I had done that week (we were always trying to paint from a photo), and Matt would pray, tell me what I had done well, and then offer suggestions for improvement. After 18 months, I decided it was the right time to stop my weekly sessions, as I felt the need to try to paint on my own, but I continue to work with Matt in a more limited way and, when I can, participate in the group sessions with some of his other students.

Even in my own overly critical judgment, the portraits I have done with Matt's guidance are quite wonderful. Some are based on real people; others are a product of my imagination. They include:

- *Frank,* an old man whose well-worn baseball cap casts a shadow over his wrinkled face; it reminds me of my grandpa (see Figure 8.1). Wrinkles are amazing. When you paint them, it is like capturing complex landscapes with hills, rivers, and occasional mountains and caves. *Who knew?*

FIGURE 8.1

PORTRAIT OF FRANK

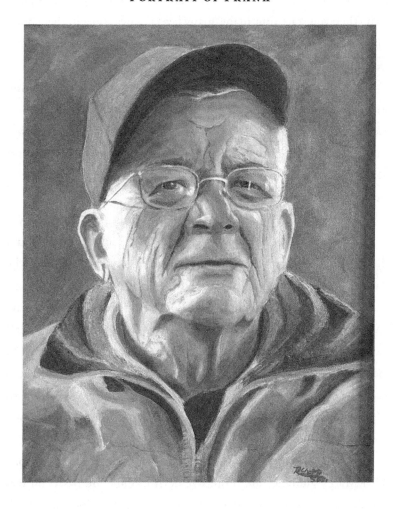

- *Ingrid and Skye* (Figure 8.2) depicts a beautiful girl with long, flowing locks of red hair (painted with pyrrole orange, yellow, alizarin crimson, and dark umber brown) seated next to her dog, a Chow Chow, whose enormous coat, paws, and eyes beckon to be stroked.

FIGURE 8.2

INGRID AND SKYE

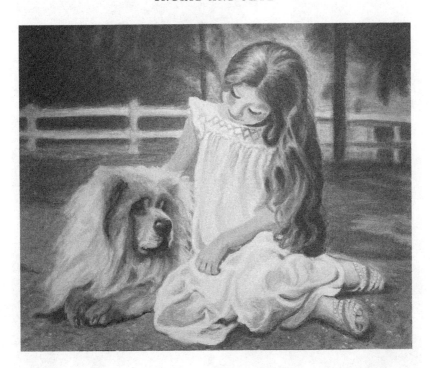

- *Nora*, a young girl who I think might be Spanish (Figure 8.3). She has flawless skin, with light gently illuminating her right side and a dress made of lace. The light on Nora is spectacular. Who knew I could do this? The sense of achievement in learning something new—especially given the recent failures of my brain—is a godsend.

FIGURE 8.3

NORA

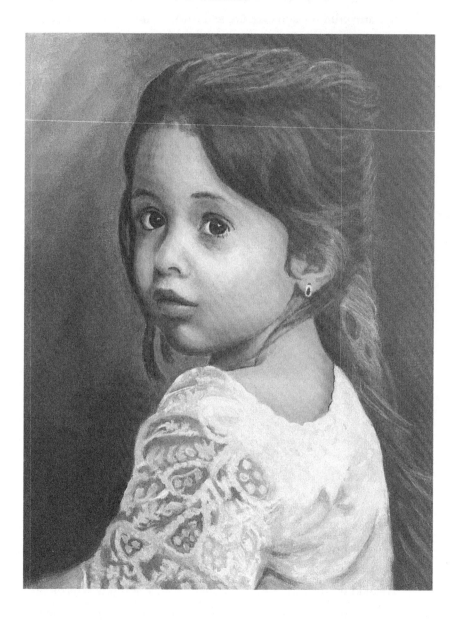

Matt taught me so many things, such as the difference between hard and soft edges, and at least four different types of blending. Matt's palette allows only seven colors, and from them one can make an infinite variety of shades and hues. I learned how to hold the brush as if it were a feather and how to paint layers on top of one another in a way that makes them, in the end, look smooth and glossy.

But, most of all, Matt taught me to see beauty in new ways. The practice of my art—as tutored by Matt—became not merely about putting paint on paper, but also seeing the subject I was painting in much finer detail. Suddenly, I would see the sky in new ways—a mixture of blues, some lighter, some brighter, some with more yellow.

Falling in Love with Faces

Through my work with portraiture, I came to fall in love with the details of faces. Older faces became so beautiful to me; I just wanted to go somewhere and sketch older people with their wrinkles, wizened eyes, and hair no longer so perfectly styled. Maybe it is my own age, but I think older faces are so much more beautiful than younger ones. Of course, this created some embarrassing moments when I could not stop myself from trying to share my newfound appreciation. One day, chatting in line with an older woman at the grocery store and feeling friendly vibes between us, I said to her, "You have the most beautiful fine wrinkles in your cheeks." Whoops! She looked at me in horror and turned away. And another time, with my daughter-in-law, I pointed out her amazing nose and said I really wanted to paint her to see if I could capture it. Luckily, she is sweet and knows that my Alzheimer's sometimes leads me to say odd things!

Seeing In New Ways

Matt led me to the practice of art that gave me the ability to see in new ways. I found a greater sense of wonder, steeping my soul in beauty. I look at a sky I once considered simply blue and now marvel at a multi-color collage of blues, teals, and greens. Where I once saw a brown stew, I now notice how the heat turns the white carrots into a lovely shade of yellow ochre. I now see the difference between the bunnies on my street and start to give them names and hope they aren't eaten by either of the two foxes, one slightly larger and more yellow-gold, the other smaller with a slight reddish-orange tinge to the fur on his back and back legs. What a delight to see with such detail! I could walk forever and dwell in beauty. I ponder, too, how just as I'm learning to see and appreciate these details in life, Alzheimer's will soon enough take away my memory of them.

As a child, my active imagination took a narrative form. My dolls would go on fantastic adventures as nurses to heal soldiers overseas or as detectives to solve the mystery of a child's disappearance. As an adult, my imagination allowed me to see new possibilities for colleges, like a library, community center, and coffee shop all rolled into one at Colgate. Painting has allowed my imagination to engage in color and shapes without specific narratives attached (see Figure 8.4). I can see all sorts of unusual shapes and imagine them colliding or combining with each other. It's not unlike the kaleidoscopes I had as a child, where I turned the dial and shapes and colors ran into each other, ever changing and enchanting. Now the kaleidoscope is in my mind.

This abstract imagination in bright colors has been noted by other Alzheimer's patients. When I asked my friend Geri, a photographer, how her art has changed as her disease progressed, she talked about seeing colors more powerfully and shifting from photographing birds to more abstract objects. And there is a bit of scientific research on artists who kept painting even after they were diagnosed with Alzheimer's. My favorite such painter is Willem de Kooning, whose greatest work (in my opinion) was accomplished with amazing colors and indescribable abstract shapes, in the last years of his life.

FIGURE 8.4
ABSTRACT IN COLORS

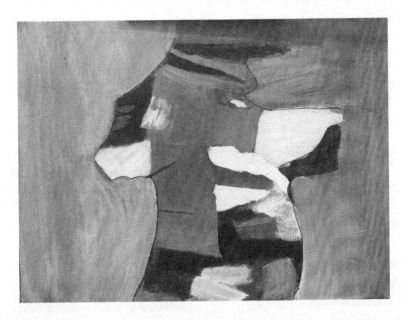

In reality, this painting is filled with many shades of reds, oranges, blues, purple, and greens, as well as black. It has been a novel experience to let colors flow through me without relying on a preconceived notion of an image.

My practice of art has fundamentally changed the way I see the world around me and find the beauty of life itself. I believe art can do this for anyone, but it most certainly can do this for those of us in the early to mid stages of Alzheimer's. The Alzheimer's Association's Memories in the Making program offers art programs for those with

Alzheimer's to paint. Some paint what they remember, as this creative work often invites memories to unfold. Others paint abstract butterflies or trees or figures.

I taught one such class in February 2023, during the period I wrote this book. I decided to teach the class of Alzheimer's patients and their caretakers how to paint abstract hearts for Valentine's Day. I painted six or seven such hearts on 10- by 12-inch canvases. Only one heart was bright red; others were pastel colors or fluorescent yellows and blues that fell off the page. I assumed people would be hesitant, so I had brought two helpers: my son, Nate, and my friend Barbara Brooks. I assumed we would have to circulate around the room and prompt individuals to paint.

Maybe because I told my own story of living with Alzheimer's, maybe because my examples were simple, or maybe because of the camaraderie among these people I had never met before, everyone sitting at round tables began sharing their stories with each other. The energy sparked.

"Everybody born comes from the Creator trailing wisps of glory. We come from the Creator with creativity. I think that each one of us is born with creativity."
—Maya Angelou

One woman painted a heart for her husband, her three children, and herself. One man, once a professional artist but now fairly advanced in his disease, got paint on canvas and then sang us a song in his deep bass voice. His wife said he had not sung for months. Another person, also fairly advanced in the progression of Alzheimer's, was able to shape a lopsided heart with various colors splashed inside and out of the heart. Nate helped him add some black to it, and his wife told me they would take it home and frame it. I didn't really provide instruction, but everyone got to hold a brush in their hand, put color on the page, and have a wonderful time.

Art lets us dwell in light and colors, even if we no longer can drive, or dress ourselves, or recall the words to describe the thoughts in our heads.

Becoming a "Real" Artist

I don't for a minute want to compare my art to some of the amazing works in museums or the incredibly gifted artists—including folk artists—at art fairs. In fact, I don't think that quality or technical skill has any bearing here. My point is that the cosmic gap between the genius artist and me or you is not as great as we imagine. Art, along with other creative activities, can be done by anyone, and anyone can be a real artist regardless of whether other people ever see the output of their efforts.

As I've come to learn, the benefits of the practice of art are endless. Among other things, it helps us break free from the confines of our left brain, and engage in practices that engage and delight our right brain. That said, I was soon to realize that yet another dimension of my life needed more attention as I began trying to live with joy in the face of an Alzheimer's diagnosis. It was the awakening of an even stronger spiritual side to my life, which I'll talk about in Part III.

Do You Need to Develop Your Left or Right Brain?

As you've seen throughout this book, my adult life prior to my diagnosis was dominated by left-brain thinking (logic, facts), though I did find joy in what I now know were activities that stimulated my right brain (creativity, intuition). If you're like me, the challenge is to find something creative—art, music, dancing, cooking, gardening, writing, photography—that will stimulate your brain just as painting did me.

On the other hand, perhaps you are the opposite of me—you have led a life that nurtured your right brain much more than your left brain. I don't have any experience with that situation, so cannot advise you specifically how to stretch your left brain other than to say you should dare to try things that don't come easily to you at first.

PART III

Lifting the Spirit and Heart

LIKE PERSEPHONE, WHO WAS snatched from the earth and dragged into Hades, I had to teach myself how to create lightness to counteract the dark forces dragging me downward. Over the course of that 18 months of transition from diagnosis to learning to live with despair and hope, fear and peace, sadness and joy, together with research and art, I began to learn to live in new ways. One of the most important avenues I've taken has led me to a place where spirituality, faith, and the experience of awe play a major role in my life, as I'll explore in the next chapters.

9

An Open Conversation about Faith and Spirituality

"We're always in the presence of God.
What's absent is awareness."

—KARL RAHNER

DURING MY YEARS OF teaching theology, I often flew around the country to give lectures and lead workshops. Inevitably, the conversations with my seatmates would turn to what I did for a living. I'd say I was a Christian theologian or a minister, which naturally led to conversations about religion and theology.

Some fellow passengers focused on the cognitive side. "Do you *really* believe all that stuff? You seem intelligent!" (As if religion were a matter of subscribing to literal truths!) Frequently, people wanted to share their own stories of trauma at the hands of a minister or priest, or of being forced to go to church with the threat of God's punishment constantly held over their heads. Or they wanted to tell me how devout they were or about their child who was not a copycat believer of the parents. Occasionally, I was asked to pray for a seatmate—right then and there. One time, on a tiny 12-seat plane flying over central

Kansas, we entered an intense thunderstorm. The plane bucked like a wild bull. Everyone grabbed hold of their seats, and I said a silent prayer of farewell and prayed for my husband and son. An elderly woman grabbed my hand and shrieked, "Pray for us; you are a minister!" (Ironically, my seatmate had just told me that her church didn't believe in women ministers.)

Plane flights were not exactly conducive to deep theological discussions; rather, the conversations seemed to just fill time (except the one about divine intervention to save the plane falling from the sky!). So I stopped mentioning the words "theologian" and "minister" and avoided having conversations with strangers about faith and spirituality. (Once I changed my career path, I would readily admit that I was an administrator in higher ed. At that point, my seatmates would just tell me where their kids were going to school or complain about the cost of tuition.)

Since my diagnosis, conversations about faith and spirituality have become common again—but well outside of academic or ecumenical spheres. Almost everyone who is familiar with my life has wanted to know how my Alzheimer's diagnosis has affected my spiritual life. And those who meet me now, when they find out that I am a theologian and minister, seem to want to talk about spirituality more than they do the recent research on drug therapies, what stage of the disease I'm in, or how my family is handling all of this. I often hear the question, "How can you believe in a God who gave you Alzheimer's?" My short answer is that I don't believe God is an angry taskmaster who "gave" me Alzheimer's.

Patients and caregivers alike often signal a desperate need to have open conversations—about loss, financial pressures, or the many decisions that have to be made at each stage of this journey. That seems to hold especially true when it comes to spirituality. Not too long ago,

I spoke over Zoom to a group of caregivers about this book, outlining my own story and what practices I employ to create joy and stay healthy. Many spoke up and wanted to know more about the practice of spirituality in relation to Alzheimer's. One man wrote to me after the session and described how caring for his wife brought him closer to God. Another wrote to say she had never thought that much about theology but had many questions now about God and religion. Opening the door to those conversations is the goal of this and the following three chapters.

That's why, in the heart of this book, I want to explain why I find great inspiration in my spirituality. I will also share some ways I spiritually deal with this tragic disease. Be forewarned that, like everything else associated with Alzheimer's—and like all discussions about religion, faith, and spirituality—there are no neat lines or boundaries. Things can get messy.

Plus, I want to underscore that what I'm sharing is just my story. When it comes to spirituality, I know firsthand that people have very different experiences, and their religious environments and personal struggles give them different perspectives to understand, deepen, or even avoid elements of spiritual connection. But still I'm hoping that reading about my experiences will help you clarify your own decisions about faith and spirituality and how they can comfort and support you.

A Theological Mis-Fit

Throughout my adult life, I have never easily fit my faith into neat categories. Others recognized this fact when I attended seminary. There, all students were given a theological diagnostic test to see if we were "fit" theologically—that is, how the ways we interpret scripture, experience, and express our faith would provide us a firm foundation for ministry.

Soon after taking the test, I was called into the dean's office. I was 20 and really scared, wondering what the heck I had done wrong. I was told that I probably wasn't fit because I hadn't scored as either a coherent liberal or conservative (in a theological sense) on the diagnostic.

Always wanting to do well on all tests, and wanting to fit in, I had a day or two of panic. What would I do if this this mis-fitness proved to be a problem? But one day as I walked across Swope Park in Kansas City (near where my seminary was located), I began to think my mis-fitness was rather delicious. Why *should* I have to choose? And what if the experience of God in the world isn't always coherent in a theological sense?

I decided to continue at seminary and eventually became an ordained minister, which ended up serving to enhance my belief that I didn't have to choose a single specific way for religion or faith to be expressed.

For example, when I served as a pastor in the United Methodist parish system in the 1970s, I quickly learned how people in the same church—with the same professed creeds and beliefs, singing the same hymns, and served by ministers trained at the same seminaries—can experience as many differences as they do similarities in their relationship with the divine. One of the first churches I served was Ash Grove United Methodist Church, a small stone church sitting in the middle of a wheat field on a dirt road in Kansas. The only members who showed up at nine thirty every Sunday morning were a group of about a dozen widows. These elderly women cared for each other: they were the Body of Christ to each other, singing their hymns, helping each other out, remembering and asking each other about their families.

Later I served two other churches, seven miles apart. Americus United Methodist Church was composed of farmers and meat plant workers. Their lives were hard, especially for those who put in long hours at the slaughterhouse in dangerous, smelly, and sordid conditions.

Yet Americus was filled with joy, with many of the people speaking in tongues (rare for a Methodist church) and reaching out to serve the community, especially children and the elderly. The other church, Calvary United Methodist, was on the verge of closure due to being located across from the largest church in town (also a United Methodist Church). Calvary was grieving, sad, and unhappy—with no mission to speak of. While Americus boomed with new members and new programs, Calvary continued to shrink no matter what anyone did.

As I've mentioned before, being an ordained woman minister in 1977 was a new phenomenon. The congregation at Americus (the congregation of farmers and meat packers) quickly decided I was sent by God and filled with the Holy Spirit. They frequently told me how fortunate they felt to have me there. In contrast, Calvary's congregation found my presence to be another sign of their impending demise. Their members did not want me anywhere near marriages or funerals, lest they not "take."

As communities, they had very different experiences of religious practice and church community. They had radically different congregations yet sang the same hymns, professed the same beliefs, heard the same sermons, and received the same pastoral care. My husband joked that one church was born *again*, and one was born *against*.

My growing appreciation for the similarities and differences in how faith and spirituality were expressed fed my determination to continue my own spiritual explorations.

Theology Expands My Understanding

After seminary, during which I served as a part-time minister in several churches, I became a full-time minister for several other churches, then eventually went to graduate school to become a theologian.

Through those diverse experiences, I got to experience worship of all different types. At seminary, I delighted in getting to know the spiritual experience of my classmates, whose beliefs spanned everything and anything. And I read works published by the church fathers, contemporary theologians (even women!), and learned about the sociology and anthropology of churches, and some of the history of Christianity. In this theological/spiritual Disneyland, I tried all the rides and went to all the exhibitions. And I liked to quote Augustine, the most important of all church fathers, "Wherever truth is, it is God's."

During my years as a student and minister, I loved the way theology opened, expanded, and guided my life. In graduate school I learned that every theologian seemed to have a distinct way of knowing God's grace. Consider the four different Gospels in the Christian Bible, the different forms of Buddhism and its many different Bodhisattvas (people on the path toward awakening or becoming a Buddha), or the many rabbinical midrashim (commentaries on Hebrew scripture). Each witness sheds a bit of light on the darkness, yet no single person can show us the full countenance of light. This makes it important that we debate beliefs and share with others the religious teachings that are important to us. Our words help enlarge our experience and help us avoid faulty action.

> "The people who know God well—mystics, hermits, prayerful people, those who risk everything to find God—always meet a lover, not a dictator."
> —Richard Rohr

My years of *study* taught me that theology helps us experience, understand, and guide our lives in a less-than-coherent and increasingly fractured world. My years of *life* have taught me that theology is only words without meaning unless we have a living experience of ultimacy—and acknowledge that, at times, it is very hard to feel ultimacy. In the same way, religion is meaningless unless one is grasped by and grasps the love of God (to use my own theological language).

All of these experiences have helped reinforce for me that all our environments and experiences are, at the same time, similar yet unique.

Spiritual Experience and the "Ultimate"

I want so much to describe my spiritual experience. I wish I could paint a picture. It would be swirls, blocks, and some lines. It would have colors of magenta and orange and blue, but also gray, drab taupe, and, of course, black—a cold, haunting black like Hades.

There would be light and darkness and shadows, but most of all the picture would be full of movement, as if to portray not a pyramid with a definite and mathematical order, but rather a lake and sky constantly meeting and changing. The problem with language is that to express reality, it also tends to follow or create order. Linear thinking, words in sentences and paragraphs, seems too neat for my spiritual experience. I find that ironic, since I am a theologian who has published multiple academic books on such topics! But what I aim to convey here is a more personal understanding of faith and spirituality, and it certainly is not linear.

I live, these days, in the world of the spirit and the physical. More than ever before in my life, I resonate with the depth of life and death, often feeling a presence of beauty and peace, but these times can turn gray and dark. A presence of "the ultimate"—a word used in religious and theological circles to represent the most basic experience or expression of a sense of universal connectedness or a higher power—seems to be with me, though sometimes that spirit lurks out of reach. The ultimate has many names, but I call it God.

Pitching a Big Tent

Throughout my life, I've found that this "similar yet unique" mantra is not just true for communities, but truer still for individuals and how they experience and express the presence of a God or ultimate power. Because my experience with spirituality and religion has been quite rich and varied—and my theology draws upon almost everything I learned—I pitch a big tent around religious experience and theology (and even Alzheimer's); I want to be open to how each person experiences God (or their equivalent) rather than try to prescribe boundaries around what is and isn't spirituality or religion.

Fred (my husband) and many others, for example, go to church to sing. I attended an Episcopalian church for a short time, and while the priest gave amazing sermons, the woman I usually sat next to perked up most when she gazed at the stained-glass windows. Over a glass of sherry (a favorite sacramental drink of Episcopalians), she told me about looking at the windows, smelling the incense, feeling the sense of spaciousness in the sanctuary, and tasting the bread on her tongue. God manifested to her through her senses.

I have so many good friends for whom ultimacy—the highest expression of the experience of God—is manifested through justice and righteousness. Of course, I have also known many who find the sense of ultimate in literal truths, in what they define as "correct" beliefs and a fixed set of boundaries on their religious experience.

My father—who you may remember likely had a severe learning disability—attended church for a brief time but left because he didn't understand the words in the prayers or the sermons and therefore could not fully appreciate the experience. In his daily life, he was shocked at how frequently self-proclaimed Christian businessmen were unethical. Dad clearly experienced, though rarely expressed, a kind of ultimate claim on him to be a good man—a calling by what he understood as

God to live his life in a certain way. But he did not share this knowledge with his family.

At the end of his funeral, after all the friends and family members had left, three strangers, dressed in rough working apparel, arrived at the church. They looked uncomfortable, even reticent, as they entered the sanctuary. I was elected to go speak to them (the role of the minister in a family). These men told me how my father had given them—and a lot of others, apparently—a second chance after getting out of jail or rehab or whatever other trials they had overcome. None of us—not my mother, nor my siblings, nor I—knew this about my dad. I was taken aback, a little surprised, and deeply proud. Somehow, learning about this grace my father had extended to others helped me to make great sense of an unspoken creed of a man I knew to be so kind and moral.

Dad's experience of what mattered to him, in an ultimate sense, was to be a good man. Though he didn't need formal religious teachings to understand what it took to be a good man, I wonder if his experience would have been enlarged by learning religious/theological language to help him name and make sense of his experiences.

As I hope you can tell from this chapter, my personal belief is that there isn't one "correct" way to experience or explain God. I am not a literalist: I don't believe every detail of every story actually happened the way it was told first orally, then in written form. The stories describe real human experience—of loss, of joy, of anger, of love. The more I studied the Bible, Quran, and other religious texts, and the more I experienced life, the more I realized that holiness and purity ("right" thinking and action) are not synonymous.

Rather, I believe that God comes to us in different ways, and the spirit of being grasped by God can as easily occur through nature, stained-glass windows, a prayer or meditation group, giving second chances to those who have experienced tribulations, or a wonderful sermon or religious teaching.

I believe our commonalities are as important, if not more important, than our differences. I tend to see the differences among us as real, and something we can learn from. I don't like narrow categories or strict boundaries when it comes to religious experience, theology, or even Alzheimer's.

Mysticism and an Infinite Union with God

I used to find it unbelievable when someone told me God was *always* present for them. It always sounded forced. But perhaps I was in the presence of mystics in those moments, and perhaps now I am having a bit of a mystical journey myself.

Mysticism is what most religions describe as an intimate union with the ultimate, the infinite, or God. Almost all religions have mystical or contemplative disciplines: meditation, prayer, pilgrimages, and, yes, even drugs to induce mystical moments. A *mystic* is "one who has moved from mere belief systems or belonging systems to actual inner experience," according to Richard Rohr, who describes himself as a Christian mystic. Hinduism and Buddhism talk about the third eye. These different descriptions transcend language and rational analysis. My mystical experience is definitely triggered easily by nature, art, and music. But with my Alzheimer's, I find that the more I am open to my "actual inner experience," the more I am able to practice a new way of seeing and being. As the mystic traditions teach, one can learn to become one with the infinite. Perhaps it is natural to gravitate toward this as one thinks increasingly about mental decline and physical death?

I think of Betty, a congregant in one of my first churches, who emanated grace. The wife of the owner of the only bank in town, she ran a small gift shop. She was a nice-looking woman, a little plump, with her hair always pulled back in a French twist. Whenever I saw her—in her store, at church, in her home where she often entertained—I felt a holiness emanating from her. Desmond Tutu, who was occasionally on the faculty of Candler when I was provost at Emory, was another who emanated holiness. But neither Betty nor Desmond Tutu was aglow with happiness all the time. I was with each one of them when they experienced health troubles of loved ones and as they agonized about the affairs of the world. But in dark days or light, they were both clearly in touch with the holy—that enigmatic ultimate that I call God.

Though it is hard to explain, I've learned we can intentionally work at being open to these moments of connection through what the Christian tradition (as well as others) calls mysticism. I used to think about mystics as being those rare creatures who lived in solitude in caves in the desert or in cloistered convents. But now I know there is a kind of everyday mysticism as well. It takes time and practice to experience it, just like learning to play an instrument or learning to paint or becoming an accomplished athlete.

My Spirituality and Alzheimer's

My own spiritual path has been a Christian one, albeit a bit non-traditional in that I have never felt confined by another person's or institution's teaching about religious experience and about the ultimate. I have learned a lot from other religious traditions, especially Judaism and Buddhism.

For me, spirituality has been central to how I cope with having Alzheimer's. I recognize that not everyone experiences spirituality in the ways I have across my life, and certainly few have had the professional opportunities I have had to learn from so many others in churches, seminaries, and college religion departments. But I do wonder if Alzheimer's doesn't lead us to some spiritual opportunities—to ask questions, to listen, to learn, and most importantly, to abide by something that is deeper, greater, and more ultimate than us? This is my great blessing now: in dark days, in gray days, and in the many days filled with light, I am in touch with God.

But living with this diagnosis, and trying to live in the light as well as the darkness, has caused me to find new resources in Christianity, resources teaching me how to lament, how to experience contemplation and joy, and how to cope with utter despair, topics I'll discuss in the next chapters.

What Is Your Experience of Spirituality and Religion?

You may already be a practicing Buddhist, Jew, Christian, Muslim, or Hindu. You may be a seeker, looking for truth wherever it is found, or you may follow other paths. I like the phrase "finding truth wherever it is found," or, said differently in the Augustine quote I cited earlier, "Wherever truth is, it is God's." I suggest only that you find spiritual resources to help you not only deal with frustration and despair, but also to open yourself to peace, joy, and connectedness. In that way, Alzheimer's can give you a small gift.

10

Crying Out to God: The Value of Lamentation

IN MY FIRST YEAR OF SEMINARY IN 1974, I served as a part-time pastor in an urban church in Kansas City. This small, financially struggling church was affiliated with several different Protestant denominations and called itself "Independent United Church." What this really meant was that various denominations funded it (though barely) to serve a new influx of poor immigrants who were not really welcome and did not feel comfortable in the established predominantly white churches. Needless to say, it was very different from the rural Kansas churches I had served up to that point.

Early in my service at that Kansas City church, I was invited to attend the wake of an Irish parishioner. The local Catholic priest had agreed to preside over the funeral service. The wake was noisy, even boisterous—a combination of crying, singing, and laughing. To my utter astonishment, alcohol was served. As people shared stories of the deceased, and as the noise grew with the amount of alcohol consumed, the crying gave way to loud wailing. It was unlike anything I had experienced before.

That year in seminary, I took classes in the Bible and had my eyes and ears open to parts of the Scripture that, if I had read them before,

I surely hadn't understood. I read about people like Moses arguing with God, disciples disagreeing with Jesus, Mary weeping, and Esther using her beauty, wits, and guile to trick a king.

How could anger, disagreement, weeping, and trickery be in this book of God? How could such negative-sounding incidents be part of people's experience of the ultimate?

I eventually learned about the act of lamentation: crying out to God, to the ultimate, about what was happening in people's lives. In the Bible, the act of lamentation (not just the book of Lamentations), it turned out, was about how people suffer and hurt, about how they felt life was unjust, about how they couldn't quite grasp the presence of God.

Learning about these concepts taught me that anger and weeping could be expressions of religious experience, too. Rage and despair were described in this sacred text. In the Hebrew and Christian scriptures I studied, much of the lamentation was about political and social destruction—often tied to evil or turning to false idols. But as I came to appreciate after my diagnosis, lamentation in the scripture is also about personal loss, about good people suffering tragedy.

Songs of Lamentation

In the middle of the Bible are the Psalms, 150 songs (the word *psalms* means songs). My heart and head connected when I read the Psalms, which I found to be an intuitive way to speak to and of God. Today, I continue to turn to the Psalms for solace, for praise, for just the right words about religious experience. I turn to the Psalms for comfort, joy, and hope. The language of anguish in the Psalms is simply without parallel and reminds me that suffering is not at odds with a connection to the ultimate.

When I received my diagnosis—when all I could think about was what experiences I would miss, the places I would not be able to travel to see, how I would become a body without a functional brain—I turned to the Psalms and read them aloud. They gave me words for my anguish and opened me up to God in the midst of my sadness.

To understand what I mean, I encourage you to read the following Psalm aloud:

> *Hear my prayer, O lord; let my cry come unto thee!*
> *Do not hide thy face from me on the day of my distress!*
> *Incline thy ear to me;*
> *Answer me speedily on the day I call!*
>
> *For my days pass away like smoke,*
> *My bones burn like a furnace.*
> *My heart is smitten like grass, and withered;*
> *I forget to eat my bread.*
> *Because of my loud groaning*
> *My bones cleave to my flesh,*
> *I am like a vulture of the wilderness,*
> *Like an owl of the waste places;*
> *I lie awake,*
> *I am like a lonely bird on the housetop.*

PSALM 102:1–7 (RSV)

The Importance of Music

I spent several chapters talking about my newfound appreciation for art as a way to develop and express my creativity in this phase of my life, but music has been important to me across my entire life. I remember singing with my sister when we were little children. I remember begging my mother for a violin when I was nine because I so desperately wanted to play music. I remember listening to country and western with my Dad driving across the plains of Kansas. I love Western classical music, rock 'n' roll, bluegrass, and so many other types.

Maybe the only way, or at least the most soul-filled way, to lament is to sing, as we cry, rant, wail. Music is often the last kind of memory we have. There is something primal about music—the rhythm and the storytelling—that taps into our emotions and seeps deep into our brain.

For me, various gospel and blues songs can give voice to my woes, my cries, my sadness. My favorite, and one I still listen to and sing, is "Precious Lord, Take My Hand" sung by so many, but most beautifully by Aretha Franklin, my favorite singer of all time.[1]

I also find that music helps me express and experience my anger—and I think we should be angry about this disease, the current lack of treatment, and the cultural stereotypes surrounding it. I don't listen to too much music written after the 1970s, but there are some contemporary songs that are wonderful for feeling and letting loose one's anger. To hear for yourself what I mean, listen to Metallica's "Enter Sandman." Even if I don't sing along to the lyrics, the music helps let the fullness of anger out of my gut.

Learning to Lament

Lamentation is not something to be ignored or vanquished. Lamentation, I have come to believe, is an important experience of love—of life, of each other, of self, of God. Lamentation is when love hurts; it's being with God in the shadows and crevices of life. The spiritual "trick" is to stay open to God in those deep cracks of life, when one is crying or angry or feeling despair. In crying out to God, there is some sense of horizon.

Having been raised never to express any emotion, especially unhappiness or pain, I had a lot to learn about crying out in grief. As I have said, I learned this early on both by encountering other cultural traditions and by reading the scriptures, especially the Psalms. Though I knew intellectually it was OK to lament, I still spent most of my life holding it back. I might have cried a bit, but rarely.

Now that I live with Alzheimer's and have studied not only scripture but also various writers and musicians, I know how to lament loudly. I now understand that lamentation is the language of loss, and loss is one of the best expressions of love. I find that though I am long past my initial anger and grief at my diagnosis, the shadows of lamentation linger.

I hate thinking of what Fred, Nate, and others will have to go through as my disease progresses. I read about or listen to the stories of caregivers when the loved one with Alzheimer's doesn't recognize them or when the patient accuses them of stealing from them or betraying them.

I speak to people with Alzheimer's who are closer to the middle stages than I am, and many tell me, "I am still alive, I am fine," even while their caregiver carries grief and anguish in their eyes. Fred is older than I am; how will he ever put up with my inevitable decline? I lament. I can't travel far anymore, and I grieve not being able to see friends in distant places one last time, to explore new places such as Scotland or old favorites like Paris. Fred and I don't talk as much about my impending doom as much as we did, but when we do or someone asks, I can see his eyes tear up, his sadness palpable. My son, Nate, and I talk a bit more about the disease, as he actively engages in serving on advisory boards of caregivers for various Alzheimer's groups. He always says simply, "It is all so hard, so very hard." I feel his grief. I lament.

Yet as I think about the loss of that which means the most to me—my husband's happiness or even one last trip to Paris together—there is an awareness of a holiness, even an unhappy holiness. Lamentation offers shelter from the lurking shadows.

Find Ways to Lament!

My best advice is that you find ways to lament—to others, by yourself, with music. Find a secluded place and let yourself scream. Get some paint and express your loss on paper or canvas. Allow yourself to lament. It means you love.

11

Abiding in Awe and Grace

WHILE TRADITIONAL EXPRESSIONS OF BELIEF in the ultimate (God) and religion have their place in my life, one nontraditional practice has come to play an increasingly important role in my spiritual life post-diagnosis: abiding in awe. Abiding, to me, means being still with my thoughts, allowing feelings to overtake me. To simply experience something in the moment as fully as possible, not thinking about what has come before or what will come after.

I can't say with scientific certainty that abiding with awe—as an experience and an emotion—has helped strengthen my cognitive reserve or improved my spiritual strength, but it sure feels that way. Let me explain.

Early-Onset Awe

Even from my earliest memories, I experienced some kind of awe, often around the sky and clouds, or a glimpse of the horizon, and occasionally around the absolute mystery of ice cream. I don't mean just enjoyment (though I especially enjoyed ice cream); I mean the experience of something greater, mysterious, something both beyond me and something to which I was connecting at a profound level.

The first person to put words to this feeling—and, ironically, to invoke God—was my paternal grandfather. I loved riding on Grandpa Chopp's lap as he plowed his field on the family farm (the original Chopp homestead) near Narka, Kansas. We had a special connection that was somehow different than I had with others. Grandpa Chopp and his family described themselves as Bohemian. The family had emigrated from the Austro-Hungarian regime and, after being chased out of New York and Chicago, found farmland in Kansas. They were proud of being Bohemian, and to this day the gravestones are written in Czech, as were the signs in the surrounding Bohemian towns. The Chopps did not trust institutions. My family believed in land, family, and "being good people," and they didn't rely on scripture or church traditions to guide their priorities.

I was thrilled to be in my grandfather's presence and proud to be helping (in a loose sense) as he drove the old Ford tractor up and down the rows. Grandpa would sweep his arm out and say, "This is God's." It was the first religious and theological statement I had ever heard, and the awe in his voice helped me to name my experience. Now I knew that this feeling I felt was somehow connected to God. I had a sense of how to name this experience with the words "awe" and "God," even though I had never attended a church. I was introduced to God, then, by a man who knew God through his fields and not through any religious tradition.

With parents who didn't speak about Jesus, the Church, or God, I found myself wanting to learn more. One summer, an older neighbor, Mrs. Martin, asked me if I wanted to go to Vacation Bible School with her. I was beyond elated: the anticipation of this thing that was so foreign to me made me quiver. I went to Bible school with her every day for a week. Not only did we learn fascinating biblical stories about Moses standing on holy ground, Jonah being swallowed by a whale, and Jesus being baptized by John (all new to me!), we colored pictures about these stories and we got snacks.

At the end of the week, I was invited to Sunday worship service. I had never attended a worship service before, and I was excited and a little scared. My mother told me I had to be very good and dressed me in my best clothes. In the middle of a service I did not understand, I saw what I thought at first was a miracle of light. An angel (on the smallish side) with flowing blonde hair rose up from the middle of the front of the sanctuary. Light surrounded her. I was abiding in awe and wonder. I gasped aloud, and Mrs. Martin gently patted my leg. It took me years to figure out I had seen a young woman being baptized. I can smile now at my childhood ignorance, but I can also still be moved by that experience of awe and God—a kind of abiding in the light.

Throughout my years as a young person, I experienced this sense of abiding in awe and grace. On my family farm was an old, gnarly cottonwood tree. In high school I would drive my faded red Ford Falcon to the farm, climb the tree, and experience a strange feeling of being surrounded by the light; I would sit in awe.

Awe and Holiness

In some ways, the word "awe" may be too limiting; at least in my experience, it doesn't quite fully capture what I experience. When I'm in a state of awe, I feel an overwhelming presence of holiness or the ultimate (what I call God) that I can best describe as "abiding in grace." When abiding in grace, awe is transformed into an experience of reverence, of beauty, of a mystery overflowing with soft power. Abiding in grace feels like being in an ongoing stream of grace, experiencing the gift of the ultimate that can be fully present to us each moment. This almost sounds silly to me, but it is my deepest spiritual truth of living with Alzheimer's, and oddly and mysteriously, it recaptures some of my very first religious experiences, nearly forgotten after all my adult years of business.

In fact, I firmly believe that it was pursuit of awe and abiding in grace that led to my religious path. During my youth, for example, I went to the Saline County Library and read what I could find about religious experience. I recall reading the sacred texts of the Bhagavad Gita (Hinduism), the Quran (Islam), the Bible and various other texts about Christianity, and the book of Psalms (Judaism and Christianity). All these books were enchanting and confusing to me at that point. As I got older, my family briefly attended the local Methodist church. I was confirmed, and I still have the Bible presented to me at that time. My family didn't stay in church long, as it didn't seem to mean much to any of us at the time, myself included.

In my early years of college, I took a class on religion and ecology. It reconnected me with the church in which I was baptized and confirmed. I became a Sunday school teacher (I can't believe a minister let me near a classroom, but I guess no one else wanted to teach the rowdy junior high class!). Eventually, as stated earlier, I switched my college major from math to religion. I was diving into learning and experiencing religion all at once. I studied Jeremiah intensely, learned about the New Testament, took some preaching courses, and got appointed in my second and third years of college to serve my first church as a student pastor. I had a strange sense of being "home" in learning the stories, in playing the role of pastor, and in experimenting with prayer, ritual, and pastoral care.

The passion for religion and connection to both God and humanity continued to grow throughout the rest of my life: in the churches I served, in discussions about theology, as a teacher and later an administrator. But as I near what is the end of my life, the religious experience that is most powerful to me and the one that I imaginatively and authentically try to expand is this sense of abiding in the awe of God's grace. Even as retirement gives me so much more time to sit and *be*, Alzheimer's and its creeping shadow make me acutely aware that time is now limited. In this paradox of having more time and less time, I seek to feel the awe that comes to me through landscapes, poetry, music, and even science (in which I am not an expert). I am not so busy with the never-ending *doing*, but instead with the fullness of *being*.

I pay attention to abiding in awe, opening myself to grace (God's grace, for me), and letting light lift me as I once saw it lift that young girl being baptized. For me, the spiritual quest is to stay in light, to dwell in that grace as much as possible.

The Everyday Experience of Awe

The tall condo building in downtown Denver that Fred and I lived in while I was chancellor at DU faced west and north to the Rocky Mountains. Prior to my diagnosis, I would jump out of bed, grab my coffee, take a quick look at the mountains, and dive into my email to get to work—at four thirty a.m. After my diagnosis and subsequent retirement, my morning routine started to shift. I began waking up at five thirty or six. Then I'd fetch my coffee, sit at my desk in front of a huge window, and wait for the sun to cast its light upon the mountains. Through the cracks of dawn I began to experience myself and the world in new ways. Time had slowed down for the first time in many decades, and I could allow myself to be, to see, to listen, to breathe.

Now I live even closer to my beloved Rockies. Each morning I see the mountains born anew—the world created again, the landscape radically reset. No quick glance will do. I soak up the stillness of the morning and study the colors, the light, the placement of the sun, the blankets of snow or the patches of sun-parched grass, the shapes of crevices and peaks, and most mornings, the ever-changing shapes and shades of the clouds. Surely, my newly developed painter's eye is helping me appreciate new colors, shapes, and other details I used to miss. After my dog, Buhdy, has finished his breakfast, we walk on trails facing west, toward the mountains. While Buhdy sniffs and enjoys more scents than any human could understand, I bask in the awe—a landscape so massive and breathtaking that I'm not sure any human can ever truly understand.

These early morning experiences of awe will not surprise anyone who knows me. Landscapes have always inspired awe for me. Fred once commissioned Randall Exon, an artist who taught at Swarthmore, to paint a landscape of the farmlands on which I was raised. Featured prominently in my living rooms for over a decade and across multiple moves, this large portrait of the rolling green Kansan hills, the clear blue sky broken only by a contrail, still takes my breath away. Throughout my life, the shores of Lake Michigan in Chicago, the whiteouts in upstate New York, the forests of Atlanta, and the lush gardens near Philadelphia have awed and inspired me. I am, I confess, an awe junkie!

Health Benefits of Awe

Dacher Keltner, world-renowned psychologist and author of *Awe: The New Science of Everyday Wonder and How It Can Transform Your Life*, uses scientific data, cultural analysis, and personal narratives to study awe, which he defines as "the feeling of being in the presence of something vast that transcends your current understanding of the world."

Awe seems to be an experience shared across cultures, environments, and traditions. But a constant theme is the notion of mystery that transcends understanding and connects us to the world and all that is in it. Awe, Keltner maintains, is good for us because it reduces inflammation in the brain—which, as I discussed in chapter 6, is suspected to be a factor in developing and accelerating Alzheimer's. So there is a clear benefit to those of us with Alzheimer's to reside in awe.[1]

Yet awe is far more than a life hack for brain inflammation. Albert Einstein once said, "The most beautiful experience we can have is the mysterious—it is the fundamental emotion that stands at the cradle of art and science."

Abiding Is Underappreciated

As I end this chapter, I want to make sure that I'm clear about how the word "abiding" in the chapter title is just as important as "awe." I always wonder if it sounds sappy to talk about "abiding." We live in a culture that has little room just to *be*: to be open to doing nothing or whatever you enjoy doing—not to produce, or work, or do the things we feel we "should" be doing, but simply to experience awe. Many engage in contemplation as an act of self-care, and I believe that contemplation and prayer are good at quieting anxiety and lessening depression.

But abiding is, for me, simply feeling still. I may be hiking, I may be painting, I may be sitting with my husband or petting my dog, and I abide. In this abiding, I experience grace, this time in which I am radically aware of the ultimate, of God. This is a bit difficult to put into words, but I suppose the point is that it is beyond words. Anne Lamott describes the moments well: "I do not at all understand the mystery of grace—only that it meets us where we are but does not leave us where it found us."[2] In these moments of abiding with grace and awe, I live fully in the light.

Learning to Abide in Awe and Grace

My best advice is that to learn to be open to abiding in grace, one has to pay attention, make time, find the activities in which you connect to the heart of God or whatever ultimate you envision. Oh, you may be doing "something" such as walking or woodworking, but in doing it, you aren't attuned to anything else: it is just you and the ultimate.

12

Fighting the
Primordial Fears

THE TOPICS I'VE DISCUSSED PREVIOUSLY—an expansive
view of faith, lamentation, and abiding in awe—are topics that occupy
my brain mainly in the daytime, including the sunrise and the sunset.

But then there are the nights, when the nightmares let loose my
fears like a torrential storm. My nightmares are vivid, with loud
sounds and a sense of falling—both primordial experiences of fear.
My dreams turn inevitably to my fears of madness and the subsequent
isolation, intense coldness, and torture—though never to death itself.
I often cry out in my sleep, and my beloved Fred awakens me, wraps his
arms around me, and draws me close. If it is near morning, when my
dog, Buhdy, is allowed on the bed (only after four a.m.; even the most
loving spouses sometimes insist on arbitrary house rules), he rushes
to lie next to my back and lick my face or my feet or whatever he can
reach. Love awakens me from my fear, though I can't say it conquers
or casts it out.

Fear can also trigger questions that hound the minds of those of
us with Alzheimer's: Why is this happening? Did God send this? Did
I cause this by the way I lived, by what I did or didn't do? Fear can

spiral into an endless processing of questions and concerns consuming one's mind.

Nightmares are common for those with Alzheimer's, exacerbated in some cases by the drugs we take. I can change my medications, meditate and pray before bed, take warm baths, and read "happy" books, but every couple of nights, the fears come back in the form of a new nightmare. That's why I wanted to include a chapter about fighting the fear.

When Nightmares Take Over

I am on a high-speed train by myself in a foreign land. I don't speak the language. I am freezing cold with nothing to eat. Suddenly, two figures in masks jump me, throw me off the train. I am in a small, dark underground cell. I am even colder, more isolated, and I am tortured slowly.

#

I find myself in a large house. I have just moved to this new place. At first, I am happy, as I have always loved moving into new houses. New experiences, new senses of myself, and fresh chances to decorate.

But this house has too many rooms. I don't know what these rooms are for. Soon the lights go out. I am lost and confused. I can't find my way. Coldness descends. Where did it come from, and why does it feel so familiar and also haunting? What I assumed were walls and windows are countless bars. Is this a prison? The howling of unearthly creatures gets louder and louder.

Some say there are universal symbols in dreams; others say their ancestors speak to them in their dreams; yet others say dreams are sheer nonsense. My own theory about dreams and nightmares is that they carry truth only in terms of how we interpret them. For me, now, with my Alzheimer's, my fear comes to me in my nightmares. I have not yet learned how to let the holiness break in and defeat the nightmare. The terrifying absence of holiness is profoundly unsettling.

Fear is a primal instinct for humans and certainly for those of us with Alzheimer's. All mammals have it as a necessary survival skill. Researchers tell us that our first ancestors had a kind of fight-or-flight reaction to the physical dangers they faced. Fear induces a biological reaction: the heart races, adrenaline flows, and senses are heightened. I notice this when my husband awakens me. My heart is racing, I am sweating, my breath is short. Fear also produces psychological responses—terror, fright, anxiety, and horror—that linger, even after I wake and know that I am safely in my own bed.

No One Teaches Fear-Coping Strategies

As a child, I was timid. Maybe it was my diminutive size, maybe it was hypervigilance in fear of my mother's anger and threats, maybe it is just my temperament. I didn't know how to understand or explain this fear. So I projected it: I became terribly scared of Bugs Bunny—whom I imagined to be 14 feet tall and maybe even a killer under all that fur! Kathy was my protector. As the oldest child in our family, she was the first in line for my mother's anger. Kathy was also larger than me and slept on the bottom bunk.

I lost that protection when I was moved to a small bedroom of my own. My bed was now next to the window, and I had only my dolls to protect me. I was scared beyond belief. My father took my hand and showed me the window screen locks, and I was somewhat soothed. His love diluted my fear, much like Fred's love now does when he holds me after my nightmares.

Fear, I think, is universal in children and adults. Most of those fears stem from earlier experiences or deeper-seated insecurities. We may mask the underlying fears so that they present to us as, say, Bugs Bunny, or they may surface in other ways. We may be genuinely fearful of poverty, suffering, murder in our streets, racism, and violence. Fear is real. We numb it through alcohol, drugs, and other addictions, through trying to embody a "macho" persona, through acting helpless and needing to be taken care of, or through whatever seems to take the edge off. But these masks do not help us address the root fears in any meaningful or long-lasting way.

The traditions I am most familiar with—Western Christianity, modern American philosophical and psychological literature—don't teach us how to deal with our fears. Too often we are told simply to breathe (good advice, but only in the short term) and to be aware of what scares us (rational, but not enough). My fear is raw and comes at night, when "logical" defenses are harder to muster and words don't really matter. It is more like a beast or demon within than a rational or linear fear.

In my waking hours, my fear is straightforward: I fear I will not recognize anyone. I am drawn back once again to the stigmatized images I've referenced before: elderly women tied to their chairs, their heads flopping, their mouths drooling, some not moving, some making motions with their hands. In the daylight, when I access my fear, I am thinking about the final stages and being like my grandmothers. Sometimes, when I'm awake, I can focus on the joy and light in my life and drive away the fears.

But at night, where there is no light, my fear loses its coherence. It becomes raw and primal. I have read a lot now about western Indigenous people and their practices of how to face fear: many Native American traditions, for example, teach their people how to summon up the spirits of the ancient ones in their dreams. I've not conquered that skill myself.

Finding Courage

Dick Nodell is my former executive coach and current thought partner and dear friend. He talks about fear as being an aspect of our nature that frightens us. He says we must learn to hear this fear as "other," as in an evil spirit or an enemy within. We must learn to push back and expel this spirit, this enemy, this otherness of terror. And, of course, this battle is not a one-time event.

I have struggled to learn the practice of expelling the evil spirit of fear, so the haunting continues. But one theologian has helped in my understanding of what it will take to fight this beast in the dark. Paul Tillich, the first non-Jewish theologian expelled from Germany for his protests against Nazism, is one of the 20th century's great theologians. As he himself described, his life and thinking were on the boundaries: he made Christians uncomfortable and the unchurched nervous by trying to bring together the secular and the Christian. A perfect theologian for me! Life, for Tillich, is always ambiguous—a mixture of light and darkness, finitude and transcendence, sin and grace. I think I have always appreciated that life is ambiguous. Modernity hates ambiguity: it wants things clear, black or white, binary, true or untrue. Perhaps this modern desire for the rational and the unambiguous is why spirituality and art have both been marginalized, seen as silly and unnecessary by so many, and rarely if ever taught in schools.

In the ambiguity of life itself, Tillich talks about faith in terms of "courage." Courage is not a word we often hear as descriptive of faith. Yet in my nightmarish fear of madness, it is the deepest and strongest word I can summon to express my faith and experience of spirituality.

Tillich argues that courage is not about bravery or overcoming fear but rather about participating in life. Human existence, according to Tillich, faces that which threatens whatever it is to *be*—for me, that's madness; for others, it's death, meaninglessness, guilt, and so on.

Courage is not about hiding, ignoring, or even minimizing our fears. It is not about rising above our reality (I *will* lose my mind to Alzheimer's). Courage involves taking up life—daring to be grasped by all that we feel and experience, by what we do and are—even as we face that fundamental threat to our existence. It is acknowledging that which is inevitable and simultaneously appreciating that which is right in front of you. Tillich uses the term "courage to be"—the courage to take life in, in its ambiguities and possibilities, in its riches and its sorrows, and be grasped by this faith.

Courage is a wonderful word. In French, the word *cœur* means heart, as if living from the heart. Latin uses the term *fortitudo,* or strength. German (Tillich's native tongue) uses *tapfer* for firm, weighty, and important. Somehow in this mix of words, the notion of facing the fears by living from the heart resonates with me. And the practice is finding the light in the cracks of the darkness of that fear. Not ignoring the darkness, not pretending it doesn't scare you—but allowing yourself to see the cracks of light all the same.

And if you think you don't have enough courage on your own, perhaps you can draw inspiration from your heroes.

Summon Your Heroes

In the mid-'90s, Maya Angelou came to Emory University and spoke at Glenn Chapel one evening. Typically, I would rather savor the words of great poets and thinkers in print or hear a recording. I find the distraction of the crowds lessens my experience and, far too often, the great person disappoints. But I knew Maya Angelou would not disappoint, and I needed to see this phenomenal woman in person. All these years later, I don't remember what she said, except her words at the end of her speech regarding *he*roes and *she*roes. I remember her saying—in that deep, knowing, captivating voice—"Summon your heroes and sheroes and take them with you. When you face adversity, when you are fearful, surround yourself with heroes and sheroes." In my own words, summon the image of those you have seen live with courage and channel their courage as you find ways to live life despite your fears.

This view of courage is a profound and spiritual way to face those beasts, to survive those lions in the den, to go into cold, dark, isolation—and still press on. I know the Christian teaching of saints is often about praying for their intervention, as if we have a God that is not quite sure of his grace or love toward us. But my own sense of the saints, whom I now love to read about, is they are heroes and sheroes who model how to fight those fears and move into the light. Saint Dymphna's mother instilled in her a deep Christian faith; after Dymphna's mother died, her father, a powerful king, descended into madness. Looking to remarry, he settled upon Dymphna, his own daughter, because she reminded him of his late wife. Dymphna had the courage to flee and used the wealth she took to establish an orphanage. She had the courage to fight his prison of madness and flee into the light.

But there are contemporary saints of courage I have known. Carrol Keeney was a member of the Americus parish I served after seminary. Actually, his wife was a member. By the time I met Carrol, his body was distorted and wracked by multiple sclerosis. He had been a prison cook and didn't have the financial resources for sufficient medical treatment. He lived in a nursing home and, frequently, in the hospital. Facing incredible beasts that tortured him, Carrol composed religious poetry all day. At night, he would recite the poems he had written in his head and then recite them to his wife. I visited him as often as I could, even as a young minister. When I was with him, I stood witness to his courage, to his living with heart. Perhaps writing this book is, for me, a way to channel Carrol. Writing on matters this personal is new—and frankly, quite scary—to me.

The Jewish theologian Susan Shapiro, a dear friend of mine since 1978, recently taught me about the song in the Hasidic tradition "Kol Ha'Olam Kulo," which counsels, "The whole entire world is a very narrow bridge and the main thing is to have no fear at all." In the Hasidic tradition, God is directing your way along that narrow bridge. Fear is transformed, as is life itself, by God as you travel this path. There are all sorts of religious practices that help you on your path. But one that is so very relevant to my own sense of the performance of courage as a way to transform (or at least cope with) those fears is the rabbinic stories in which dancing and singing bring about the miracle of transformation. Martin Buber, a well-known Jewish philosopher, tells one such story:

> A rabbi, whose grandfather had been a pupil of Baal Shem Tov, was once asked to tell a story. "A story ought to be told," he said, "so that it is itself a help," and his story was this: "My grandfather was paralyzed. Once he was asked to tell a story about his teacher and he told how the holy Baal Shem Tov used to jump and dance when he was praying. My grandfather stood up while he was telling the story and the story carried him away so much that he had to jump and dance to show how the master had done it. From that moment he was healed. This is how stories ought to be told."[1]

Before I sleep into my nightmares now, I tell myself shero and hero stories, in hopes that I can enact them in my dreams. While I don't dance and sing before bed (I do dance and sing a lot at other times), my sheroes and heroes, I believe, have the power to dance and sing my beasts away.

Living from the Heart

Spiritual times are not all times of light. Most of the stories we tell are about great religious figures and about despair, suffering, torment, and even death. God runs through all these stories. For me, the dark times are times of intense fear, and now they almost always arrive in my nightmares. Fear is a primal reaction to real or imagined threats. And what is more threatening than death? Well, sometimes that fear of losing my independence feels more threatening than death itself. Fear is like a wild beast within that rears its head without any explanation or even an identifiable trigger.

This growing darkness is the hardest for me to deal with, and my path is getting narrower. But to live from the heart, to face the inevitability of death, to vanquish my beasts—that is my quest. These stories of heroes and sheroes, and my husband's loving embrace, return me to love as moonlight shines through our windows.

Some people tell me they have "conquered" fear, and perhaps that will happen to me eventually. Though I hold out little hope it will. For me, I am striving to face fear spiritually, to take it in and live with courage, with the heart to move through it. The darkness of fear, when I take it in with courage, can lift into the light. Again, it is hard to explain with words. What helps me is the stories of others: as Maya Angelou calls them, the heroes and sheroes. I love reading about the saints, for they all had this courage—itself a connection to the ultimate—to live through those fears, and for many of them that included martyrdom. I have my own everyday sheroes and heroes.

Develop Fear-Fighting Strategies

As I discussed in this chapter, few of us have been taught during our lives how to fight fear. Those of us with Alzheimer's no longer have the luxury of believing that fears will dissipate in the daylight or, on their own, loosen their hold on our dreams at night. Though I wish I could give you a list of actions proven to reduce fear, I don't have the answer. And it seems likely that no one strategy will work for everyone.

So my advice to you is to start developing your own strategies for fighting fear. Pay attention to what gives you comfort. Are there things that decrease the frequency or intensity of fear, or at least can help you recover more quickly? What gives you courage?

As you learn what works for you, please share! I love collecting stores of new ideas, so I hope you will share with me your story. And also how you practice courage in living with Alzheimer's.

PART IV

Reframing Orders as Gifts

I HAVE NEVER BEEN GOOD AT taking orders. I have always been independent, but I also just don't follow directions well. And it's been that way all my life.

When I was in the fourth grade, I was proud of being a Girl Scout. I loved wearing that green uniform, belonging to a group, and earning those badges to sew on my sash. I was a quiet, good Girl Scout—until one day the leaders of our group took us to ride bikes on a decommissioned airplane runway. Our leader wanted us to ride in single file. This made no sense to me given the width of the runway, and I was sure that riding side by side would motivate us to go faster and farther. So I broke out of the line and rode up beside our leader and gave her my suggestion. Like Medusa, the Greek monster who could turn brave heroes into stone by looking at them, my scout leader's glare could have made me and my bike a permanent granite statue on that airstrip on the Kansas prairie. One thing led to another, and I was kicked out of Girl Scouts for not obeying that order.

Every time I had a teacher, a coach, or a trainer who barked out orders, I found it harder to learn. I could be left alone to learn, I could be supported to learn, but hard orders didn't work for me. But an Alzheimer's diagnosis comes with "doctor's orders" that must be obeyed: diet, exercise, stress management, social and intellectual engagement, and restorative sleep.[1] Orders, orders, orders. Face it: this is a terminal disease. (I know what the end will look like, and it is literally the stuff of my nightmares.) Now, upon learning that my worst fears would become reality, I was ordered to give up some of my favorite foods: cheese, ice cream, french fries, and yes, sweets. I was ordered to work out *two hours* a day. I was ordered to have social connections. I was ordered to sleep, as though I'd be able to sleep on command.

I have always chosen to live a fairly healthy lifestyle. Though a child of the '50s, when girls didn't play sports, I have always loved to walk and bike. I stopped eating fast food so long ago that I can't even remember going through a McDonald's drive-thru. I have worked out for years, largely to keep my stress at bay, and being a fairly social person, I have loved to see my friends and be around people. Needless to say, being an academic kept me intellectually engaged.

But now, what I thought were life choices had become orders that affected nearly all aspects of my life. At first, it struck me as counter-intuitive to continue and expand my healthy lifestyle. Shouldn't this be the time, as I face decline and death, to kick back, quit exercising so much, and eat whatever I want?

The short answer is no. These lifestyle interventions are backed by lots of research. To be clear, these doctor's orders will not prevent you from getting Alzheimer's. They will not keep you alive forever. But the research shows they may slow the progress of your symptoms and greatly improve the quality of your life. And for those who have not been diagnosed with Alzheimer's, this type of healthy lifestyle may delay the onset of symptoms.

Pardon me for repeating myself, but I think this is important. Tempting though it may be to give up in the face of such an awful diagnosis, these interventions can potentially prolong the "good years" by slowing the progression of Alzheimer's.

For me, the lure of having more quality time with family and friends was a compelling enough reason to take my doctors' advice seriously. But stubborn as I am, I had to reframe their instructions and commands. So long as I had the imagined Medusa scout leader giving me orders, it would never work.

Time and time again in my life and career, I have reframed problems into possibilities. But how could I reframe these doctor's orders in a way that would create a win for my body, my soul, and my temperament?

If you've read the earlier chapters, you won't be surprised that I found my path forward by drawing upon an analogy to a Greek myth—specifically Perseus, the Greek god who beheaded Medusa. The young Perseus was ordered to do the impossible and slay Medusa in order to save his mother. Legions of brave heroes had been turned to stone, and their statues populated the entrance of the cave where Medusa lived. But Athena, Zeus, and Hermes, some of the most famous of the gods, looked upon brave Perseus with favor. Athena gave him a polished shield, while Hermes gave him winged sandals that would allow Perseus to fly.

Having received these gifts, Perseus approached Medusa with his back turned toward her, using the shield covered with mirrors to view Medusa's reflection. He used Zeus's unbreakable sword to cut off the head of this terrifying creature. The sandals of wings allowed him to fly away.

In short, these gifts allowed Perseus to triumph with courage, purpose, hope, and yes, joy. Perhaps I could think of the "orders" I was receiving as "gifts" that would slash into my fear of madness. Perhaps I could be inspired to see my life in new ways.

I now reframe myself as Perseus, adorned with gifts that will save—or at least maximize—life itself. The following chapters focus on three such gifts that I'm currently focused on: exercise, nutrition, and sleep.

I try not to focus on what I can't do, but rather on the opportunities I have been given that will ensure I can live to the fullest even as I face my death. Maybe these gifts will slow my symptoms from developing; maybe they will just make me feel better as my symptoms progress. But these are gifts to help me live well, and may do so for you as well, as you'll read about in the next three chapters.

13

Exercise, Buhdy, and Being Fit

THOUGH I HAD BEEN ACTIVE all my life—and absolutely love hiking—I didn't get serious about exercise until I was 55 years old. I have kept up with exercise and being active ever since. Still, even for me, being told by my neurologist that I had to exercise *two hours* a day came as a shock. I feared having to spend that much time exercising would turn my love of activity into hate. So how could I reframe that order to exercise more as a gift? Naturally (for me), I did some research then set about developing exercise habits that would work for me. What I discovered and how I look at exercise now is what I'll discuss in this chapter.

Exercise and Alzheimer's

Exercise is critical for living well with Alzheimer's. Every book and article I have read on lifestyle intervention stresses the importance of exercise. The body needs to be as healthy as possible to slow the deterioration of the brain. Many common conditions—including heart disease, diabetes, and obesity—can be risk factors for Alzheimer's, and they need to be addressed and moderated. Exercise helps fight inflammation in the brain and, as I experienced, keeps stress at bay.

Neuroscientist Wendy Suzuki, in her TED Talk "The Brain-Changing Benefits of Exercise," notes that exercise is the most transformative thing you can do for your brain for three reasons.

First, exercise has an immediate effect on the brain by increasing levels of neurotransmitters like dopamine, serotonin, and noradrenaline. Her lab demonstrated that performing a single exercise activity can improve your ability to pay attention and your reaction time for up to two hours.

Second, Suzuki says exercise has long-lasting effects on increased attention span, controlled by the prefrontal cortex (the front-most part of your brain, right behind your eyes). That means the benefits of exercise on the prefrontal cortex continue throughout the day. Ongoing exercise should mean that I have a stronger prefrontal cortex to pay attention.

Third—and most important to me—is that exercise increases the size of the hippocampus, where long-term memories reside.[1] A great deal of research has linked exercise, especially aerobic exercise or "cardio," to increased volume of the hippocampus.[2] David Brown, author of *Beating the Dementia Monster*, explains how this occurs:

> It turns out that exercise promotes the production of a protein that participates in the "neurogenesis" process—the generation of new brain cells—and it apparently helps repair them as well. The protein is called "brain-derived neurotrophic factor," or BDNF. It is believed that BDNF regenerates brain cells by promoting stem cells in the hippocampus to form new neurons.[3]

As Suzuki says, "So with increased exercise over your lifetime, you're not going to cure dementia or Alzheimer's disease, but what you're going to do is to create the strongest, biggest hippocampus and prefrontal cortex so it takes longer for these diseases to actually have an effect."[4] Reread that quote because it may well be the biggest motivation for lifestyle interventions. If it means that I can hold on for a little longer to those memories of my family and friends, the memories of my travels and people I have met along my careers, and the memories of hikes and strolling—to remain myself for extra months or years—I want to do all I can to support my hippocampus!

Brain Benefits I've Experienced

As I write this chapter, I'm happy to report that my reaction time is still quite good, though my attention span is awful. I get an idea for this book or I need to respond to an email, and by the time I walk into my office, which is 20 feet from my living room, I can't remember a thing. I am even starting to forget which way I am going when I run an errand, so I often have to turn around to get to where I am headed. To help take advantages of the impact of exercise, I try to sit down to work on this book or undertake other complicated tasks immediately following a dog walk or workout session.

How I Became a Midlife Athlete

My life changed in an important way when I was the president of Colgate University nearly 20 years ago. It is an active place, and the typical student is extroverted, fun, and athletic. A Colgate faculty member,

Ellen Kraly, was a survivor of breast cancer and decided that she and I should hike Mt. Baker in Washington state as a way to raise funds for breast cancer research. Mt. Baker is less than 11,000 feet in elevation, but it has glaciers and is a steep climb. The last 1,000 feet is sheer ice!

The women's basketball team agreed to do much of our fundraising, and the project became an all-school activity. Trainers in the recreation center agreed to help Ellen and me get into shape. I was 55 at the time.

The decision to train for this hike would likely have surprised the people who knew me in my youth. I had never thought about myself as athletic. I was little, a bit awkward, and I had no muscle. I was the nerdy kid who lacked confidence in my physical abilities. I was always the last picked for any type of game in gym class. In junior high, my gym teacher taught me how to keep score for basketball games and fencing matches, which I believe was a tactic that would prevent me from competing!

Long before I came to Colgate, however, I discovered that I would rather hike than do almost anything else. I was first introduced to hiking when I was 18, and I have hiked my way through life. I have hiked almost every mountain chain in the United States and strolled across hilltops in Europe and Asia. I even like tramping across prairies, something I did long before I was 18. There is something about being in nature that makes me feel one with the universe, that lets me experience the peace of God. Smelling the freshness of the pine or the strength of the sage, seeing the beetles and butterflies and bees, and observing the trees, the sky, the soil. Plus, I like the physical effort of lifting my body up the steep, rocky slopes where I live or those lush, rolling green hills in Ireland.

So it was with optimistic enthusiasm that I embraced the training needed to hike Mt. Baker with Ellen. Our trainers had us in the gym at six o'clock every morning, and on days we weren't in the gym, we hiked the hilly upstate New York campus with 30 to 40 pounds in our backpacks, usually in the form of gallon jugs of water. Lumpy, awkward, and designed to throw us off balance, carrying the jugs prepared us for the 50 or so pounds we would carry on our climb.

Being an athlete taught me so much. I liked being on a team—and Ellen and I were very much a team as we helped each other train, prepare, and hike. I enjoyed the shared sacrifice and victories. Though I had always been disciplined about getting work done, I learned to apply that discipline to the training. I would make myself meet Ellen at what used to be a ski hill at Colgate that had a 370-foot rise (or drop, depending on your direction) in elevation. We'd be carrying those backpacks laden with water jugs in the freezing cold, and hike four or five times up and down the hill. Some days I failed; I had to quit by the third trip. But I tried again day after day. This gave me a whole new appreciation for the athlete who trains and trains no matter what the weather, her mood, or how tired she is.

Eventually we did the hike on Mt. Baker. In the end, I couldn't make it all the way to the top, though Ellen did. But that was nearly inconsequential because the process itself was fulfilling. After all that hard work, I was an athlete.

That experience and my total of seven years at Colgate, on top of my love of hiking, taught me the sheer fun of working out and enjoying physical challenges. Colgate, in this and other ways, taught me to find the athlete within me. I kept up the rigorous exercise routines by hiking with backpacks and climbing mountains in Vermont, New Hampshire, New York, North Carolina, and Colorado. I joined more "team" efforts, most of them dedicated to raising money for causes such as cancer and multiple sclerosis. I worked with trainers while at Swarthmore, at DU, and now in my retirement. I learned about muscles, days off, multimodal movements, various types of cardio, and how to stretch.

I even learned to kickbox, which I think, next to hiking, is the single best exercise in the world. For me, all this exercise during my academic years was fun—a stress reliever and a way to burn off the calories from the near-constant eating a university president does while attending functions to meet with donors, faculty, students, and others.

Enter My Canine Companion

Dr. Hudson's prescription to live with joy and exercise *two hours* a day called for a combination of cardio, strength building, and choreography (exercise with a mind–body connection such as ballet, kickboxing, some types of barre, and yoga). I then realized that I needed to tend to the athlete within me more vigorously than ever before, calling upon the winged sandals of Perseus.

I trusted this doctor and realized these orders were a real gift, if a challenging one. I knew I could do strength training and some type of choreography for an hour a day, but the other hour was going to have to be cardio. And an hour a day on a treadmill might work for some, but I simply could not do it!

Fortunately, in Colorado I can get this extra hour of cardio in by indulging in my favorite activity of hiking. About six months of the year, when conditions allow, I hike the foothills in and around Denver. On nice days without snow, I venture even farther afield by heading out to the mountains. I love the thought that hiking plays an official role in fulfilling the prescription to be healthy and live with joy!

That first summer after my diagnosis, I hiked at least five days a week. If I wasn't driving or being driven somewhere up into the Rocky Mountains, I hiked Mt. Falcon, a peak to the southwest of Denver not far from my home. It has a steep 1,800-foot incline over the course of a 1.8-mile trail. It's a great training hike, always challenging and guaranteed to include lots of birds, critters, trees, wildflowers, and plants to observe. Until recently, I generally hiked alone, so I appreciated that the trails were well known to me and full of other hikers. My sister or a friend would sometimes accompany me, and we could talk during the tramping or afterward over lunch.

But six months of the year I cannot hike, as the foothills and mountains are covered in snow and ice. Plus, I knew early on in the diagnosis that I wouldn't always be able to drive myself to a trail. And, as I age, I know that I probably won't be able to do extensive hiking even four days a week. Walking around my neighborhood, alone, for an hour or so a day would not be inspiring. I would need a reliable companion.

The perfect solution, of course, was to get a dog. Our current location, Anthem Ranch, is a community with 48 miles of trails and proximate to multiple dog parks, other trails, and great open spaces. I had to work a bit to convince Fred, especially because I decided I wanted a puppy. I had not had a puppy since I was 21, as all my other dogs were older rescues. But I had watched my son and his wife raise countless puppies, and I longed for the utter cuteness, love, and boundless energy that a puppy brings. I liked the idea of watching a puppy grow up, and I was curious about how I could train the puppy to be a companion and, in part, a service dog. Plus, if I got a breed that needed lots of exercise, I would get the gift of cardio exercise, too.

So the search began. After extensive research, I settled on a pomsky, or arctic spitz, which is a medium-sized dog that is a mix of husky and Pomeranian (not yet a formal breed). Sounds odd, but absolutely beautiful. They have energy and a fun, quirky personality like the husky, but are loyal and loving like the Pomeranian. I found a great breeder of this mix, and within a few months I had my puppy. The breeder had told me this was the best-tempered dog of the litter and sent me one picture that made him look totally Zen—like a little Buddha. I thought it would be great to have a little Zen Buddha in my life, so I named him Buhdy.

As of this writing Buhdy is two years old and is a well-behaved, adorable dog who loves lots of walks and occasional slow jogs. Buhdy has a wonderful temperament and was relatively easy to train. Most days, we put in an hour of vigorous cardio exercise.

But, of course, Buhdy is far more than a workout partner. His companionship, playfulness, and emotional support bring me joy and add to my overall wellness. Caring for his needs helps me to stay alert and feel a sense of purpose and responsibility after my sudden retirement.

The study of service animals for those with Alzheimer's is just beginning, and I believe that there is incredible opportunity for dogs to provide more than just companionship. Domesticated dogs have long been used to provide assistance for those with blindness, deafness, post-traumatic stress disorder, diabetes, epilepsy, and more. As anyone who has had dogs can attest, dogs are acutely sensitive to their person's physical and mental well-being. Research has shown that dogs help keep people calm. Almost anyone who has had a beloved dog companion knows how relaxing it can be to cuddle with the dog after a long day. Even just petting a dog with slow, soothing strokes brings peace.

Since many people with Alzheimer's lose their ability to follow a routine, dogs—who thrive on routine—can be trained to help keep their people on schedule. A dog can be trained to bring things to people with limited mobility, to make sure someone doesn't leave the house, to alert others if their person falls, even to lead a person home when lost. When I say "home" to Buhdy on one of our walks, he knows how to take me there. I haven't needed to rely on him for that yet, but it's a comfort to know he will be able to get me home if someday I can't remember the way. Several times I fell in the Colorado snow, and Buhdy stood guard over me and barked until someone noticed.

My Exercise Gifts

The gift of Buhdy, of canine companionship and service, gives me great joy. In fact, all the gifts of exercise—whether hiking, lifting weights, or ballet and barre—bring me joy, just as Dr. Hudson prescribed. Sometimes, as I walk with Buhdy or lift a weight or hold on to the barre as I stretch, I picture my hypothalamus growing and my prefrontal cortex full of new connections.

What Will Get You Moving?

I feel fortunate that I discovered a love of hiking early in my life and a love of exercise when middle aged, long before I was diagnosed with Alzheimer's. Yet even for me, it has been a struggle to put in as much time as is needed to keep my body and brain healthy. I also know that many people with Alzheimer's simply cannot be as active as I am because of other health issues.

So my best advice has to be to consult with your physicians about what you can and cannot do physically. If at all possible, find something you love to do that will get you moving—walking, hiking, dancing, canoeing, whatever!—and do as much of it as you can. Many Medicare programs now include reimbursements for gym memberships, so you can explore that option as well. Just keep fighting to be as physically fit as you can possibly be. The brain benefits are worth it!

14

Cherishing Nutrition as Lifesaving

I LOVE ICE CREAM. Have loved it for my entire life. So one of the hardest orders I struggled to reframe as a gift was to give up ice cream and other fatty and processed foods. Changes in diet are never easy, even when you know there is a good reason for doing so. In this chapter, I'll talk about my history with food and what it took to change a lifetime of eating habits.

Memories of Ice Cream

Most people I know agree that "ah, yes, ice cream tastes so good!" But for me, ice cream is more than just a food. It brings back some of the happiest memories I have.

My first memory of ice cream was with my father and Grandpa Chopp (the same grandfather who introduced me to spirituality and creation). Grandpa Chopp would occasionally drive down from Narka, Kansas, to where we lived in Wichita. I am sure it was an enormous adventure for this man who rarely left his farm. Grandpa Chopp loved baseball, so when he visited, my dad and I would spend hours watching baseball with him on our black-and-white TV with rabbit-ear antennas. One day, at the conclusion of a game, my dad announced we were going to get ice cream. They put me in the back seat of my dad's big turquoise-and-white 1954 Chevy 150 sedan with whitewall tires, and off we went. I was with the two people who were the absolute loves of my life. Two men with whom I felt totally safe. We drove for miles, or so it seemed, and stopped aside a small wooden structure with picnic benches outside. My dad bought us cones, and we sat on that bench, me between my two protectors, and ate that luscious ice cream.

Ice cream was about love, but it was also about resistance and independence for me. My mother had enormous problems with food. I still don't fully understand the reasons for her obesity or for her need to have absolute control over the food the rest of her family consumed, though I assume the two were related. We were forbidden to open the refrigerator and get anything to eat. All of us, including my father, ate what and when we were told to eat. But when I was in high school, my dad and I started rebelling. Ice cream, in the late '60s, was pretty cheap at 59 cents for a half gallon. My father and I would wait until my mother had gone to bed, then get the ice cream out of the freezer. We would stand there—like two naughty children, big spoons in our hands—gobbling marble fudge vanilla, butter pecan, Neapolitan, or sometimes black licorice ice cream. Of course my mother would curse us the next day. Her temper was real, and the fallout could be unpleasant. But either my dad or I would just go buy more!

I continue to love ice cream as my favorite food on earth. Sweet, creamy, and evocative of so many wonderful memories. But I no longer eat it.

Ice cream, like other highly processed foods, is horrible for the brain. The dairy in ice cream is like death itself. The high fat content encumbers the very connections in the brain that need to be free. The sugar leads to explosive growth of inflammation, that great enemy of the Alzheimer's-afflicted brain. OK, my language here is admittedly hyperbolic. But I have had to demonize ice cream so I can view the ban against eating it as a gift rather than an order. I let myself have some healthier types of ice cream on rare special occasions. But now, after a couple years of daily abstinence, I no longer miss it. Oh, I still love the cold, sweet taste of ice cream, but it is the memories I cherish most. And I can tell myself, quite truthfully, that *avoiding* ice cream is what will help me hang on to those cherished memories as long as I can.

Food and the Brain

As a child of the 1950s, I ate lots of newly available processed foods. For people like my parents, fresh off the farms, it must have been amazing to go to the store and buy cheap white bread, overprocessed bologna, "cheese slices" that probably wouldn't qualify as cheese, and cans and cans of baked beans (the kind flavored with ketchup, brown sugar, and loads of salt). We still had farm food like fried chicken, peas in a thick cream sauce, corn, mashed potatoes laden with butter and gravy, and cakes galore. Even with a mother who controlled every morsel, this was not a brain-healthy diet. This diet was what so many in my generation grew up on.

At some point, the culture woke up. Long before my Alzheimer's diagnosis, I became aware of the need to eat more vegetables, avoid fried foods, and drive past, rather than "thru," those fast food places. Like many American girls, and especially one whose mother was very ashamed of her body, I was often restricting my calorie intake. At least I knew to diet with foods that were by and large healthy—with the exception of diet dressings and diet sodas, which I would later come to find were not at all good for my brain either. Of course, before my diagnosis, I would balance my diets with ice cream whenever I could.

By the time I was 45, I had already begun to think of food as fuel for the body rather than comfort or indulgence or the lack of it as punishing calorie deprivation. After my Alzheimer's diagnosis, I wanted to understand what food did to the brain. Even though I had thought of myself as a brain with a body attached, I never truly considered how the body affects the health of the brain itself.

Dr. Hudson strongly encouraged me to investigate and follow the MIND diet.[1] A version of the Mediterranean diet, MIND could be a significant factor in prolonging my good years. Although Dr. Hudson told me that I could occasionally "cheat" on this diet, I didn't want to do that without understanding the repercussions. So I investigated why food was so important in terms of brain health and how I could reframe this type of diet (which was not one I followed at that point) as a gift. My research led to a series of small revelations:

- Fat is incorporated in membranes of the neurons, and according to *Diet for the MIND*, "the *type* of fat determines how well neurons transmit signals to other nerve cells in the brain or to your muscles and other organs."[2] Fatty fish, like salmon, keeps our neurons flexible and helps with neurotransmission.

- Complex carbohydrates provide fuel and energy to keep the brain and other organs functioning.

- Antioxidants, found in berries, vegetables, and other foods, fight the formation of free radicals, which are chemical forms that are highly reactive. An overabundance of free radicals contributes to many chronic and degenerative illnesses, including Alzheimer's. (I'll talk more about free radicals in chapter 15 on sleep.)

- Most of us know that protein builds muscle, but it's easy to forget that the most important muscle of all is the brain. As we age, we need much more protein to keep our muscles, including the brain, strong. (Exercise requires us to eat even more protein.)

There's so much more to be said about what food does to and for the brain. How do I manage to see all this as a gift? Once again, research was the bridge to my reframing. Although it's not a particularly scientific notion, I began to imagine my brain in cosmic terms, with the forces of good battling the forces of evil. Maybe this is another instance of me being overly dramatic, but as Cheryl Mussatto, a clinical dietician, puts it, "Foods are either brain sustaining or brain draining."[3] If all the horrible processed, fried, and nutrition-drained canned foods of my youth were Kryptonite, then healthful proteins, complex carbs, dark green veggies, and berries would be my superpower foods.

So as I buy and prepare food, I ask myself, "Good for my brain or bad for my brain?"

Embracing the MIND Diet

Diets are always a bit controversial among even the experts. Some insist on a strictly plant-based diet, while others claim that certain animal-based proteins and some types of fish are critical in limited quantities. Some say no to eggs, while others say eggs are a great source of protein. Some say avoid all alcohol, while some say a glass of red wine per day may actually be good for you. It's tempting to look at the conflicting advice, determine that these experts can't even agree, and shrug your shoulders while enjoying the foods that you love. But we all know that despite the quibbles over some of the specifics, some approaches are objectively more healthful than others.

The MIND diet that my neurologist recommended is probably one of the easiest diets to follow, as it allows lean chicken and turkey and can be adapted for the occasional trip to a restaurant. Though many restaurants are starting to add more vegetarian and vegan dishes, the offerings are usually quite limited. The MIND diet brings together the Mediterranean diet and the DASH (Dietary Approaches to Stop Hypertension) diet. The MIND diet focuses on the brain-healthy foods from both approaches, as well as evolving research on nutrition and dementia. The MIND diet adapts a 15-point "score-card," though I never keep score and instead prefer to draw from its general guidance:

> Earning the top MIND diet score of 15 means eating at least three servings of whole grains, one serving of vegetables, and one glass of wine each day; in addition, it means eating leafy greens nearly every day (at least six times a week) nuts most days of the week (at least five times a week), beans about every other day (four times a week), berries twice a week, poultry twice a week, fish once a week, and using olive oil as the main oil. Finally, it means limiting as much as possible the foods that aren't great for brain health, but definitely consuming less than 1 tablespoon of butter or margarine a day, pastries and sweets fewer than five times a week, red meat fewer than four times a week, less than one serving of whole-fat cheese each week, and fried fast foods less than once a week. Meeting each of these requirements earns one point each, adding up to a possible score of 15.[4]

The MIND diet is fairly lenient as diets go. I like that it focuses on foods *to* eat and denounces without outright prohibiting bad foods.

Food as Adventure

One thing I ended up loving about the MIND diet was that it gave me an excuse to learn about some new foods from cultures from Asia, India, Africa, and Latin America—all of which include more fish, beans, and a wider variety of whole grains than I was used to. I also embraced the growing trend of vegetarian recipes and the wisdom of groups such as Seventh-Day Adventists and Sikhs, both of whom emphasize plant-based foods.

My New Relationship to Food

I ended up embracing the MIND diet recommended by Dr. Hudson, though without much enthusiasm at first. And I do not ever count the points recommended in the MIND plan, though everyone will find different approaches to be more or less effective.

Now, I cherish food as something that helps me to live longer and better—to prolong the good years. I find joy in knowing that every bite I taste is a gift to cherish rather than a step toward hastening decline. To find that joy, I avoid red meat almost always, limit my sweets to at most once a week, and eat berries and nuts daily. I enjoy the adventure of making great lentil soup, black beans and rice, vegetable curry, and other new, easy, and often cheaper ways of cooking. I limit myself to what my neurologist called the SMASH fish: salmon, mackerel, anchovies, sardines, and herring. A twice-a-month trip with a good friend to a sushi restaurant is my new version of going out for ice cream.

I have also changed my whole mentality of when I eat. In the years when I was a university president I lived by the motto "never eat alone," both because it allowed me to meet with more people each day and because food provides a ritual of social connection. When I met with a staff person over lunch, we were a bit more relaxed and I found out more during those times than in the hurried weekly sessions at my conference table. Students loved a free meal, and we generally filled the time with laughter as well as conversations about what was on their minds. I often learned about faculty research over lunches or small dinners. I formed deep and important connections with alumni over dinners, lunches, and occasional breakfasts. I enjoyed going to the fancy, now-closed restaurant at the Four Seasons in New York City and people watching or meeting donors. The Yale Club was so beautifully formal, and I lunched with some of the most interesting donors, who could discuss religion and politics at length. My favorite places to meet donors in Philadelphia were those amazing Italian restaurants on the south side of town, some with only two or three tables.

What I now realize is that the food played a minor role in all those meals. It was the ambience and the people who were important to me; I honestly didn't pay much attention to the food. And that habit of not paying attention to the food—mindless eating—became a habit. A few meals I savored, but more often than not, eating was incidental to talking and connection.

Now I have a mindfulness and spirituality around consuming food. I eat slowly and deliberately, tasting the many complex flavors. I think about where it grew or was raised, I give thanks for the food, for those who raised it, and how it can contribute to my brain. My husband has numerous GI problems, and the diet I follow, full of roughage and complemented by lots of spice, is not for him. So we eat different foods while sitting together. The pleasure is being with him, not in eating the foods he eats; foods that are better for his digestion are often not so good for my brain. When I do go out to eat, which is not too often anymore, I cherish the opportunity to break bread with a friend or family member.

In short, food now is another of the gifts I'm using to help me maintain as much of my brainpower as I can for as long as I can. I like thinking that food cultivates my brain. It adds protein to build brain cells. I'm tending to my brain's neurons and connections with those bits of broccoli, Brussels sprouts, and many berries. Getting rid of those devilish free radicals by munching on my nuts and dried soybeans. The cosmic battle in my brain is won by every good bite I eat and every bad bite I avoid. Well, 90 percent of the time anyway!

Think about Diet

Dietary choices are unique to every individual. I can tell you from my experience that I've been able to follow and even enjoy the MIND diet, but I'm not in a position to say it's the best diet for every person. Just be aware that your food choices will affect your brain's health. Educate yourself about the options out there and find something that will help you preserve and extend your good years as long as possible. That's the path I've chosen.

15

The Healing Luxury of Sleep

I TALKED EARLIER ABOUT MY lifelong relationship with sleep and how little of it I ever got or thought I needed—until the months leading up to my diagnosis. I have come to learn that my pride in not needing much sleep was a false pride, and that sleep has benefits that the brain craves. I'm hoping that by explaining my background more fully in this chapter, you will no longer downplay the need for sleep, as I did, and instead use my experiences as an impetus to change.

False Pride in Not Needing Sleep

For most of my life, I didn't enjoy sleep. When my mother made us take naps when my sister and I were small, I would not sleep. I used the time to imagine playing new games with my dolls, building castles in the yard, and riding my bike. As I grew older, waking up in the middle of the night allowed me to be with my father, or enjoy playing with those dolls or reading a book. The habit continued throughout my adulthood. Being able to get by on four to six hours of sleep a night gave me the equivalent of an extra day each week to work, to be with my son when he was little, to get things done. I was even proud of the fact that I got by on so little sleep, thinking I had cultivated a superpower of sorts.

Now I regret that sense of false pride. The lack of sleep was dangerous, probably hurting my brain and making me more susceptible to Alzheimer's. Studies have shown that people who don't sleep much (fewer than five hours per night) are twice as likely to develop dementia.[1] I don't blame myself for my Alzheimer's. We don't know what causes this disease; we only know there are correlations.

But truth be told, even if I had known that statistic, it probably wouldn't have convinced me to change anything. From childhood until the last year before my diagnosis, I couldn't sleep. Stress, an overactive brain, too many problems to solve—it would all wake me up, even when I was exhausted.

Decades of Segmented Sleep

When I was provost at Emory, Fred and I lived in a Mediterranean-style townhouse, filled with light and large rooms. The bedroom was on the top floor, the living space on the middle floor, and my study in the basement. I loved that study. I had built bookshelves on a long wall. I had a lovely black desk large enough to spread out all my papers and books. I sat in a blue leather desk chair that I had bought because it seemed fit for a princess working at her desk. Next to a window was a favorite green-and-blue striped sofa with a large footstool for propping my feet. The basement window had a large casement on which someone had painted sunflowers against a pale blue sky.

Around one a.m., I would creep down the stairs so as not to wake Fred, turn on the lights, and be in my own world. Many nights, I would find other senior colleagues who were also awake and sending emails (as I discussed in chapter 2). We would discuss the problems of the moment and start planning next steps. I would read documents, compose emails, or begin some big project. I would return to bed around four o'clock and either sleep or, equally likely, just toss and turn.

This middle-of-the-night phenomenon didn't occur just at Emory. At Yale, I would get up, go down to the main floor to a study that countless deans had used before me, and try to figure out tough problems. At Colgate, in a beautiful study that I designed to include built-in bookshelves and a wood-burning stove, I would sit at my desk in front of a window and plan all the wonderful building projects and scholarships and other programs we would launch. And so it went at Swarthmore and DU. Different offices, different issues, but always the same busy mind, working when most other people were sleeping.

At some point I stumbled upon some information about "segmented sleep" and learned that Benjamin Franklin and many other leaders enjoyed some time in the middle of the night. They would go to bed at eight o'clock, sleep for a few hours, get up for a few hours, and then go back to sleep. I decided that segmented sleep was a necessary leadership trait, justifying and taking pride in what I viewed as segmented sleep.

What I now know is that segmented sleep was a phenomenon in preindustrial societies that didn't have artificial lighting. For people living in those times, nighttime wakefulness was not a time of anxiety and stress (as it is for many people today). They ate, did chores, made love, relaxed, took cold-weather baths (perhaps by simply opening the windows), or gathered with others over a warm drink.[2]

What I had was not this preindustrial break in the night, but a type of chronic insomnia called middle insomnia, or middle-of-the-night insomnia, which is a type of insomnia that can contribute to heart disease, diabetes, strokes, and of course neurological disorders. There should certainly be no pride in having a sleep pattern that could contribute to those health problems.

The Brain Benefits of Sleep

What I've come to learn after my diagnosis is that sleep is fascinating. At first, during sleep, the heart beats slower, muscles relax, body temperature drops, and brain waves slow. I like to pause on each of those elements and imagine them—as if I am simply floating in the air, totally relaxing. These periods of sleep are when bones and muscles, including the brain, are repaired.

Then REM sleep happens, and the hard work begins. According to neuroscientists, the brain activates various regions. The brain is cleaning itself of free radicals. The Cleveland Clinic website paints a colorful image of free radicals:

> When the steps are followed precisely, molecules work in concert to help keep you healthy. Like a line dance gone awry, though, if one molecule slides to the left while the other slides to the right, crashes are inevitable.
>
> Enter free radicals, the molecules with the potential to crash your party, if left to their own devices. "Free radicals are missing an electron from their outer shell. That makes them unstable, so they go and steal an electron from the molecules in your skin cells, or from your blood cells or from wherever they can. That causes damage to surrounding cells," DiMarino explains.
>
> Thinking back to the dance, free radicals are the belligerent friend who'll grab anyone in arm's reach to do-si-do.[3]

This image hit home in part because of a bad recent experience I had with line dancing. After moving to my current home near the foothills outside of Denver, I thought I would take up line dancing. It is popular here, with six or so different levels of instruction and all sorts of fun-sounding groups. I had always loved to dance and had taken various classes in modern dance and ballet. I figured I would have a great time learning steps, singing songs, and stomping and clapping. When I got better at it, I knew I would make one of the "dance teams" and perform at various places. The best team performs at Denver Nuggets games. I could see myself there, getting the crowd to sing and clap with the other members of the team. So I joined up for the beginners lessons. I also knew this would be great for my brain. Over the first three sessions, I was humbled by the new limits my Alzheimer's had imposed. I couldn't learn the dances. I stumbled all over and literally grabbed a woman before I fell. I myself had become a free radical!

In short, sleep is very good for us. It allows our brains to be cleansed and our cells to be repaired. Sleep is a gift that keeps on giving in so many different ways.

Napping as a Resistance Movement

Sleep is personal, but in this day and age of stress and anxiety, it is also political. We need to sleep. Sleep is, indeed, good news. While I was writing this ode to sleep, for example, I learned about the Nap Bishop. Tricia Hersey was, like so many in our culture, stressed and exhausted. An epiphany of sleep occurred, and now she is known as the Nap Bishop. She provides collective places to sleep, which rather reminds me of my son's preschool that had naptime during which all the children slept on their special rugs, alone but also together. Hersey started a spiritual movement that, as she says, is also "about imagination work, justice work."[4] The Nap Bishop calls her work a resistance movement.

The Gift of Sleep

I have mentioned that about a year before my diagnosis, I started sleeping much more. Suddenly, I couldn't wait to go to bed. Whenever I could, I would go to bed around eight thirty p.m. and sleep until five thirty or six a.m. I had to change my workout times because I could no longer get up at four thirty a.m. On the weekends, I slept until six thirty or seven a.m. and took naps. I enjoyed it. I was amazed, though I was worried I was not getting as much work done. Fred, who loves to snuggle, thought it was fantastic. Neither of us thought it might be a sign of anything other than aging. I never would have guessed that an increased need for sleep would become, thanks to my wonderful family doctor, the first sign that something might be wrong with my brain.

Sleep was the doctor's order that was the easiest for me to reframe as a gift. Even if I resist it, sleep, as my husband says, overtakes me. I now sleep when I need to, Fred on one side and Buhdy on the other. Even when nightmares come, and I am awakened by my husband and licked by my pup, I fall back into the good news of sleep.

Take Sleep Seriously

If you are already a good sleeper—hooray! If sleep is more of a problem with you, please consult your physician. There are medications that can help you sleep. Taking a little pill is much better than not sleeping. Your brain will thank you. Pleasant dreams.

PART V

When I Feel the Most Me

HOW DOES ONE DESCRIBE the notion of *self*? To be human is to be unique. Science tells us that we each have unique DNA. Certainly, even if aspects of our history may overlap with that of others, we each still experience our individual self in our own unique way. We are often defined by a temperament that may hold considerable consistency over the years. The theologian in me might focus on the unique spiritual experience, the educator would answer through the lens of distinct learning styles, and the armchair psychologist in me would answer in terms of psychological traits. Even how we come to understand ourselves is a journey unique to each of us.

But I prefer a shorter answer: **we are what we love doing and being**.

In the book *Before I Forget*, the late model, singer, and restaurateur B. Smith described music as her most essential purpose and passion:

> But I am still serious about singing: Just because you have Alzheimer's doesn't mean you can't sing . . . I am not going to forget the tunes I love, that's for sure. I'll remember those tunes my whole life. So that's my plan, and I'm sticking to it. I'm going to work for Alzheimer's and I'm going to sing.[1]

In short, singing made B. Smith *B. Smith*. For me, I am most *Rebecca* when I am actively engaging in three areas of my life: the pursuit of justice and doing what is right; finding community with a shared and meaningful mission; and sharing time, love, trials, and triumphs with friends and family. These are the areas that make me happy, integrated, full of purpose and passion. This is not to say there are no other areas of my life that I love: hiking, art, music, and reading certainly enrich my life. I hate to think of the day I won't be able to do those things. But justice, community, family, and friends have been the deep sediment that grounds me, allows me to grow and blossom, and makes me *me*. These are my deep and abiding passions. They are still with me, and they still nurture me.

I am fortunate that these most essential elements of my life ensure that I remain socially and intellectually engaged. The tremendous temptation in Alzheimer's is to withdraw. Part of this is the depression that often attends Alzheimer's, and part of it is that these forms of engagement take a lot of energy. What nourishes me and makes me *me* requires lots of energy and effort. I tire easily now, and I have to pace myself carefully—something which does not come to me naturally. (As Dr. Hudson, my neurologist, once explained to me, every day my brain only has so many "beans" to expend, and a long social engagement uses a lot of beans!)

In the following chapters, I'll talk about my ongoing efforts to engage in the truest sense of myself:

- My justice and advocacy work, now focused primarily on Alzheimer's awareness. It seems to move at a snail's pace, though I know it is urgent.

- Creating and supporting community. This works comes in bits and spurts, much of it now online, where once it consumed me full time and mostly in person.

- Tending to the garden of my friends, weeding out a few, and caring deeply for the closest ones, but with less regularity than I once could devote.

Engaging in these three areas is truly when I feel the most me.

16

Justice and Advocacy for Alzheimer's

I AM NOT SURE WHEN MY SENSE of justice first emerged. My father, as did his father, believed that doing the right things was both a first principle and the North Star. My dad rarely spoke of others with contempt, but he detested some of the corrupt contractors and subcontractors with whom he had to work. I remember him not understanding why there was such racial prejudice, since, for him, if a man worked hard and lived rightly, the color of his skin didn't matter. My father wasn't of a generation where one had easy access to knowledge about systems of oppression, unconscious bias, or structural racism. For his era, though, he judged people by how they lived in terms of ethics and hard work. My dad's ethical foundation was impossible for his children to miss, and we all grew up with his motto to "just do the right thing."

That philosophy has been a mainstay of my life ever since I was in high school and continuing through to this day as an Alzheimer's advocate. Let me show you why it is such an important aspect of *me*.

A Sense of Ethics

Ethics, for me, became a drive for justice when I was in high school. Coming of age in the 1960s, I saw the riots on TV. I read whatever I could about the systemic injustices against Black Americans, Latinos, and Indigenous peoples. I watched how the few Black students were treated in my school. A few of these boys were idolized as basketball players, but they were relegated to the back of the room in social studies, where they were largely ignored by the teacher and by their white classmates. I dated a Native American boy for a short time in high school. Brad was beautiful and sweet, a wrestler who loved cars. His mother was raising him by herself, which was unheard of in those days. My parents supported this relationship, but many at my school, including the vice principal, did not. The relationship ended for different reasons, but I never got over the experience of so many disapproving stares, comments, and attempts to pressure me into ending the relationship.

The high school I went to was very much a part of the so-called traditional culture of the rural Kansas community in which it was situated. Only rarely would a teacher mention what was going on in the country in terms of the fight for civil rights. I was hungry for more information and for someone with whom I could talk about these issues. A friend invited me to a youth group at her Presbyterian church, where the young associate pastor was an activist. I had found my people. I came to assume that Christianity, justice, and the mystical were all deeply connected because that is how this young man presented it. I had no other frame of reference.

But I was in seminary when I began to read about liberation theology, a type of theology that weaves together biblical teachings of justice with the experiences of injustice in the world. My life's calling emerged. I read the works of Gustavo Guttiérez, a Latin American theologian working against the terrific economic and structural oppression of the poor, and Johann Baptist Metz, a German theologian who imagined a political-mystical theology of hope. I knew I wanted to be a pastor and promote this dimension of Christianity that wrote and spoke from, to, and about those who were not in the center of power, but rather on the edges of society (see sidebar). After studying Rev. Martin Luther King Jr. and other civil rights activists in the US, my life's work became driven by the conviction that "Until All Are Free, No One Is Free."

God in the Margins

One of the underlying themes in my experience of faith is that I have been particularly drawn to the concept of what God calls us to do in terms of justice and mercy: I see very clearly the faces of God in those on the margins of society.

Activism comes in all shapes and forms, and I ultimately chose to express mine through the vocation of teaching and writing. I wanted to teach theologians and future pastors how to help proclaim and live into the reign of God. At the Candler School of Theology at Emory, I was hired to teach systematic theology, which I think of as discerning God in the world of our current experience, as well as feminist theology. At that point in my life, I had not read many books in feminist theology. As one of the first women ordained in the United Methodist Church in Kansas, I had my own experiences of being told no, being paid less, not being listened to, and worse. But now I was asked to interpret Christianity through the experiences of women. Given the advances of birth control, the needs of many women to earn money, and the changing structures of marriage and family, we needed and still need new narratives of what it was to be a woman, especially for those women who found themselves working, single, or raising children. The prototypical white American housewife, depicted so well by June Cleaver in *Leave It to Beaver*, no longer worked for most people. Indeed, it had always been unrealistic even for most white women, let alone everyone else. Christianity could be a resource for these new narratives, but only if Christianity itself was freshly reinterpreted, just as it had been countless times through the centuries.

After I shifted from teaching into administration, I continued my concern for justice and liberation for all. I was always focused on expanding access to those who historically had been excluded from the academy, but also educating those who had economic and social privilege to use their knowledge and skills to make the world a better place. I was being *Rebecca* when I worked with first-generation college students, when I created scholarships for low-income students, when I expanded support programs for students with inadequate preparation for college or for students who had learning differences. I felt immense satisfaction when business students learned about the inequities and possibilities in economic markets or when social work students were trained to empower the disenfranchised to get on their feet and to gain their voice.

Ironically, one of the last efforts at justice that I undertook had a direct impact on my life today. Allow me to explain.

Going Public to Advocate for Alzheimer's

In December 2019, I was awarded the Knoebel Institute for Healthy Aging's very first "Knoebel Prize." The Institute was quite new back then; it was in the planning stage when I had become chancellor five years earlier, and I had the pleasure of hiring its first director, Lotta

Granholm-Bentley, whom I have referenced earlier. (In addition to her guidance that helped me understand my diagnosis, Lotta helped me to build that bridge between the despair of Hades and the light of living on earth.)

The Knoebel Institute's interdisciplinary mission combines scientific research, the arts, and the professions to study healthy aging and also to engage the DU and the Denver communities in how to age well—that is, with dignity, wellness, and intentionality.

From the start, I was an enthusiastic supporter of the Knoebel Institute. I frequently attended research sessions on how robots could help with dementia; I even once conversed and danced with one of the robots! I talked with the faculty who were researching the development of biomarkers for early disease detection. I went to programs to engage the community, including one on Tai Chi. I loved that the Institute was drawing from resources across the university to help people enjoy and live well in the last phases of life.

The need for this kind of institute was clear, too. I knew that vast numbers of the baby boom population were beginning to retire, and I had a hunch that they weren't going to be content merely golfing and playing bridge as many of their parents had. Also, given that my own mother and so many of my friends' parents had died from or were experiencing neurodegenerative disease, I liked that most of the research would focus on the brain.

Throughout my administrative career, I helped start many interesting interdisciplinary centers to address possibilities and problems, from the future of liberal arts education to the future of democracy, but this particular center filled me with a special joy. DU would help people in Denver and contribute to research that could help millions more. Why shouldn't senior citizens benefit from the incredible resources a university has to offer?

At the time the Knoebel Institute was launched, of course I never would have predicted that I would soon need the kind of research and education it provides. By the time of the award dinner—eight months after my official diagnosis—I had been contemplating whether I wanted to be more public with the fact I had Alzheimer's and not some vague "complex neurological disorder." I had gone to a dinner sponsored by the Alzheimer's Association where a man with Alzheimer's spoke. He inspired me to realize that I could do the same thing: I could be helpful to others in my condition, and I could continue to be engaged in justice work, even if that work was just to fight against the stigma that Alzheimer's carries. I wrote my acceptance speech, but I could not bring myself to write about my own diagnosis. I was afraid to go public, even as I started to realize the potential upside to doing so.

As my husband and I drove to the event, I told him I might disclose that I had Alzheimer's. Everyone in the room had surely read or heard about the public announcement the previous summer about why I was resigning, but few people knew it was Alzheimer's. My husband said simply, "Make sure you are ready."

The banquet took place in the beautiful open auditorium on the top floor of the Daniel F. Ritchie School of Engineering and Computer Science at DU. The ceiling looks somewhat like a mosque, with beautiful architectural lines leading the eye upward and magnificent light pouring into the space. The room was packed with friends from the Institute. The program began with the awards, and I received the first of the two awards. Lotta said kind words about me as one of the founders of the Institute, gave me the award, and invited me to say a few words.

I stood up that night, looked at a group of people I knew would be supportive, glanced up to the heavens, and put away the remarks I had prepared.

I explained why DU had created the Institute and how proud I was of its work. I explained that when the Institute started, I didn't realize

I would so soon be a possible direct beneficiary of its educational and research mission. I explained that I had been diagnosed with Alzheimer's and while it had taken me awhile to share the news publicly, that night and that crowd made the right moment to do so. Everyone stood. Many were crying. I asked them to sit. I went on to talk about the need for research, for policy change, and equally important, the fight against the stigma of Alzheimer's. I pledged myself to this cause.

I knew that in however many years I had left, I had to work against the stigma, to do all I could to make sure doctors were testing and diagnosing this disease, to support the research and to actively work for policy change.

The day I stood up to receive the Knoebel Prize, I outed myself as one who has Alzheimer's. When I vowed to work for the cause of research, fair treatment, and education, I was being true to myself. I was engaging in social and intellectual engagement just as my doctor had ordered.

In the months that followed, I became active in the Alzheimer's Association of Colorado. I led a team for their annual walk to raise funds for research, wearing a blue flower. If you're not familiar with this practice, the Alzheimer's Association sponsors walks around the country each year to raise funds for Alzheimer's research. These events are joyous and fun—with balloons, bands, vendors, swag, and even free food.

Central to these walks are big paper flowers. Everyone picks at least one big flower to carry. Alzheimer's patients like me carry a blue flower. Most carry a purple flower (to symbolize that a loved one has died of the disease), a yellow flower (to signify being a caretaker), or an orange flower (in support of a future without Alzheimer's). The crowd gathers before the walk, and everyone waves their flowers. Right before the walk begins, a white flower appears on stage to represent that someday there will be someone walking who will be the first person cured of Alzheimer's. The crowd cheers madly, and the walk begins. Thanks to the Alzheimer's Association and the many other groups and individuals who raise funds to support research, I believe that someday that walk will be filled with many white flowers.

Will I Ever Carry a White Flower?

Some of those Alzheimer's patients carrying blue flowers hope and pray that they might be among those someday carrying a white flower that would symbolize they have been cured of the disease. I don't have that hope. Perhaps because of my age or perhaps because I am too much of a realist, I just don't think it's likely. But, really, I want it to be a younger person—someone who is 41, who just got a diagnosis of early-onset Alzheimer's. They have the most to gain from treatments and cures.

Still, the white flower symbolizes to me that people with Alzheimer's must live well and do what we can to delay the progress of the disease. Because a cure may be found, especially given the research frontier scientists are now exploring, and none of us knows when that might happen.

My involvement did not stop with the walks. I gave the association two of my paintings for their Purple Gala auction, plus Fred and I agreed to be interviewed for a video of our experience with Alzheimer's, and we were the guest speakers for the auction that year. After COVID restricted in-person gatherings, I attended events and meetings online.

Though I had promised myself I would never again serve on boards after my professional career, I eagerly broke that promise for the chance to sit on the board of the Colorado chapter of the Alzheimer's Association. I also spoke on several radio programs about my experience with Alzheimer's. What had led me to that first time to speak out at the Knoebel Institute dinner gave me a new sense of purpose, leading me to engage more and more.

Voices of Alzheimer's

After one of my radio interviews, Geri and Jim Taylor contacted me. Geri was diagnosed with Alzheimer's in 2012, and with her husband, Jim, became a national leader in the movement to educate the public about the disease. Geri and Jim were and still are tireless in their efforts to fight the stigma of Alzheimer's, to push for increased research funding, and to fight against the injustices in the health-care and Medicare/insurance systems that deprive Alzheimer's patients of sufficient treatment. Jim suggested that they gather a few of us with Alzheimer's together to provide support to one another.

Though I knew a number of people with Alzheimer's, I didn't know anyone else who shared my desire and ability to advocate and work for justice in relation to this disease. Either most of the people I knew hadn't been diagnosed in the early stages of Alzheimer's, as I had been, making it difficult for them to be activists and advocates, or they had just been diagnosed and needed to continue to work and were scared that their employers would find out and fire them for one cause or another. In sum, most Alzheimer's patients I knew were either incapable or felt they had to hide their diagnosis. I agreed with Geri and Jim that those of us who could needed to band together to work for everyone.

Our group was a community of support, allowing us to get to know one another and form a band of brothers and sisters. Almost immediately, we knew we wanted to speak from the perspective of those living with Alzheimer's, or in Jim's case, the perspective of someone caring for a patient. Thus, Voices of Alzheimer's (VoA) was born.

Though there are many organizations filled with individuals working to fight this disease, the Alzheimer's Association is the major player. Its funding for research and educational support is legendary. Every year, it issues a report entitled *Alzheimer's Disease Facts and Figures*, which ought to be required reading for every primary care physician, neurologist, or person touched by Alzheimer's. Other organizations—including Us Against Alzheimer's, Being Patient, and Dementia Minds—all work for the cause of ending Alzheimer's disease.

But at that time there was no organization that played an advocacy role for those of us living with Alzheimer's. We wanted VoA to be that organization. We wanted to fight the stigma that each of us had experienced and that is so common with Alzheimer's. We wanted to consult with scientists, doctors, and pharmaceutical companies about our experience, putting a face to what is too often an invisible disease. Most of all, we knew we wanted to fight public policies that discriminate against those with Alzheimer's.

Over the course of the next year, we incorporated Voices of Alzheimer's as a nonprofit organization with a board of directors, half of whom are living with Alzheimer's. We raised funds, garnered professional support, and formed alliances with other groups working on Alzheimer's. We describe our distinct role on our website:

> We want to catalyze a political and social movement on behalf of millions of families affected by Alzheimer's and other cognitive illnesses to drive policy approaches to improve prevention, treatment, and care.

Medicare and Alzheimer's

Much of our efforts at VoA have focused on the Centers for Medicare & Medical Services (CMS), the agency that administers Medicare. Medicare is the primary (and often only) health-care insurer for people over 65. It has been extremely slow to cover diagnostic and treatment procedures for those with Alzheimer's in the same way it covers those with cancer, heart disease, and other medical problems. For instance, PET scans, invaluable in diagnosing and monitoring the progress of Alzheimer's, have been limited to only one per lifetime and only if you are in a CMS-approved clinical trial. Very few patients fit this draconian limitation, so almost all people who need a diagnostic PET scan are not covered. This limitation is so unlike what occurs with other diseases where doctors can order the necessary diagnostic and monitoring tests necessary.

Medicare has a history of discriminating against those with Alzheimer's. After Aduhelm—a monoclonal antibody, or mAb, drug I discussed in chapter 6—was approved by the FDA, Medicare announced it would only provide coverage for those in clinical trials, a restriction that eliminates most of the people who would qualify for the drug. Furthermore, Medicare announced it would not be covering future mAb drugs, thus announcing before FDA consideration that drugs such as lecanemab and donanemab would never be funded. What? This is the first time in history that Medicare announced it would not fund drugs even if the FDA approved them. The FDA has the role to approve drugs; Medicare is to fund them so that patients have proper access.

This made our collective blood boil in the VoA. It was unprecedented for the CMS to refuse to cover drugs that the FDA approved for Alzheimer's or any other disease. There is not a single neurologist employed at CMS.

The unjust, discriminatory decisions will likely rob Alzheimer's patients of their remaining days, weeks, or years before they truly lose themselves. This decision could cost families millions of dollars because it means that patients will likely spend more time in expensive memory care units or full-time care at home by family or other caregivers.

I, my colleagues in VoA, and Alzheimer's activists and champions across the country were furious. The only reason ever given for the decision not to fund these FDA-approved drugs was that CMS said they were uncertain whether the medications would be effective in the real world (disagreeing with the FDA for the first time in history). We wondered: Were there other reasons? Would these drugs be too costly for Medicare in its opinion? Was it because most of the more troubling symptoms show up primarily in the elderly? Is it because there is no cure in sight and the drugs only prolong life or even just offer the delay in the onset of symptoms?

The decision made no sense! CMS covers payment for expensive treatments that extend life for anywhere from a few months to a few years in the case of other diseases. CMS has never suggested an age limit on disease treatment. And the mAb drugs don't seem any more expensive than aggressive treatments for various types of cancer.

To pour the proverbial salt in the wound, Medicare cited the cost to cover Alzheimer's drugs as one of the two reasons for the 16 percent increase in Medicare part B premiums in 2022 (the other being the depletion of funds due to COVID).

VoA fought back, joining forces with the Alzheimer's Association, Us Against Alzheimer's, and other organizations. The Alzheimer's Association and Us Against Alzheimer's did a terrific job of prepping representatives in Congress to grill CMS Director Chiquita Brooks-LaSure when she appeared before committees. Members of our organizations marched in the streets, we wrote letters, and we undertook enormous social media campaigns. VoA hosted die-ins across the country, where protestors lie down in public places to represent those who are losing their lives to Alzheimer's. In my dreams and hopes, a national movement was born!

CMS changed its decision. For the drugs with accelerated approval, clinical trial participation will be the only way a patient will have CMS drug approval. For traditionally approved drugs, patients will only have access if their physician is willing to use a registry. No other FDA-approved drug is treated this way. Currently the registry doesn't appear to be extremely burdensome, but it is still a hurdle physicians and patients face.

Progress was made, though it is a bit restricted. We are all grateful, but we are also aware there is a long way to go to make sure all diagnostic tests and approved drugs are covered, as well as forms of care.

The implications of CMS's short-sighted decision to refuse these treatments were enormous. Millions of Alzheimer's patients who could and should have had these treatments were denied the opportunity to extend their functional lives. Families were overburdened sooner than necessary, with the economic, physical, and emotional toll rapidly compounding. How many patients or their families can afford the estimated total cost of $400,000 for Alzheimer's care? How many caregivers could be expected to provide 24/7/365 care for those in the last stages of Alzheimer's, especially since the patient will likely be agitated, wandering, and unable to feed or care for themselves?

Implications for research are also enormous. Will pharmaceutical companies continue to invest funds to research drugs that might be approved by the FDA but not covered by Medicare? Or will these companies decide to put their resources into other diseases that are more profitable just because CMS has decided they are more important than addressing Alzheimer's? If CMS can discriminate against Alzheimer's based on cost to the agency, what other diseases could suffer the same fate?

Fighting the Stigmas

Though Voices of Alzheimer's is primarily focused on CMS, Medicare, and the historically unjust and ill-conceived decisions around funding Alzheimer's research and drug treatments, our fight for justice will include other battles. Surrounding and underneath all our work is the fight against stigma. This fight once again reminds me of the monstrous Medusa and the way that Perseus eventually slew her:

Medusa was depicted with bronze hands and wings of gold. Poets claimed that she had a great boar-like tusk and tongue lolling between her fanged teeth. Writhing snakes were entwining her head in place of hair. Her face was so hideous and her gaze so piercing that the mere sight of her was sufficient to turn a man to stone.[1]

Think of *stigma* as the snakes, the fangs, the tusks that turn the stigmatized—Alzheimer's patients like me, and perhaps you or your loved ones—into stone. But, as with Medusa, the monstrous and harmful stigma surrounding Alzheimer's disease must be slain. What are these harmful stigmas—these monstrous snakes? They are the false impression that Alzheimer's equates to madness; that a diagnosis means instant mental incapacity or imminent death; that even patients in early or middle stages of the disease can't make their own decisions; that getting too close means one will "catch" Alzheimer's, or at least be forced to confront that which they implicitly believe is hopeless.

How do we remove the power of these monstrous stigmas? What would it look like to behead this particular Medusa? Remember Perseus. Armed with the gifts the gods had given him, he found Medusa's reflection in his shield, which allowed him to get close enough to her so he could cut her head off—before being turned to stone. Confronting the ignorance of stigma and prejudice also is best done indirectly. Saying "that is wrong" about a person's ill-informed statement may shut that person up for the moment, but the next time you are not around, they will say it again. Knowledge, education, and information are the equivalent of Perseus's sword, shield, and winged shoes. They are the tools we can use to indirectly fight Alzheimer's stigmas.

Fighting that stigma—getting people to understand that there are millions of us with Alzheimer's, that we're still *us*, and that we deserve to be seen as fully human—is the mission of this book. Indeed, it is the mission of the Voices of Alzheimer's and fundamental to the work of so many organizations dedicated to fighting this disease.

Continuing the Fight

When I told my son that I had publicly shared my diagnosis and would devote myself to supporting its treatment and eradication, he said, "Of course you will, Mom. That's what you have always done."

My son has always known me as someone who cared deeply for justice, for ethics, and making the world a better place. It took me some time to work through my fear of disclosure—and to combat my own biases. Only once those barriers were conquered was I willing to share my diagnosis and become a public advocate for those of us with Alzheimer's. Fighting this fight is helping me be me.

How Can You Advocate?

I have chosen a very public path of advocacy through the nature of my work with Voices of Alzheimer's and my willingness to speak on podcasts and be interviewed for videos, and even writing this book. I hope some of you reading this will speak openly about the disease and its effect on your life, on what has changed and, equally important, what *hasn't* changed.

Even if you aren't as public as I am, I encourage you to talk with your family and friends and acquaintances. Every little step will help us build a better understanding of Alzheimer's among those of us affected by the disease and the people who support us. Our words and actions can influence the scientists working to find a cure and change the hearts and minds of the public at large. Please join in our fight however you can.

17

Creating Community

I DON'T KNOW WHERE I BECAME so committed to the notion of cultivating community. Perhaps it was in the rural churches I served. I watched how people cared for each other, coming together to celebrate or mourn, to care for the elderly in their community, to help raise each other's children, to worship together.

I have personally benefited from this community-oriented mindset. As I've mentioned before, I was one of the first women ministers in Kansas. It was in January 1972 that the United Methodist Church in Barnard, Kansas, received a call that their new part-time minister would be a woman. Women didn't serve in churches at that point in Kansas. Not yet ordained, I could not officiate marriages, burials, or baptisms. I had not been raised in the church and had little idea what it took to keep even a small rural church going. Fortunately for this congregation and their new minister, this church was a community filled with people who loved their church.

The people of that church stepped forward: they taught me, they loved me, and they served in all sorts of ways they had never before imagined. When I left the church to go to seminary, we all reflected on how the church was stronger than ever because they had seized the opportunity to imagine and grow in new ways, together.

That experience in 1972 drove home for me how much I relished the connectedness that comes from having a community of people working together. It was the birth of the second component of what makes me most *me*.

Developing a Sense of Belonging

When I taught Christian theology at Emory, I was frequently asked to lead Bible studies at local churches. I loved to hear what people thought of various biblical texts and how to use the text to help people find God. Although I loved the deeply intellectual conversations I had on campus, these more personalized conversations with congregants often felt more relevant to people's everyday lives.

In 1987, during Lent, the time leading up to the observation of the crucifixion and resurrection of Jesus, I was asked to lead a men's Bible study at a local Episcopal church. I had never led an all-men's Bible study, nor had I taught a class with just men in it, so I was interested to see what the dynamics would be.

I was a very good Bible study teacher, and I never failed to create spirited and warm conversations. I would always begin the first session by taking time to let people get into a creative, open mindset, awakening them to the spirit in our midst. I might ask them to introduce themselves by what kind of car they would take Jesus for a drive in. Or I'd ask them to think of the last time they felt themselves to be standing on holy ground and to describe the colors, the temperature, the sights, and so on. Then we would take turns reading the scripture, where I would make comments and ask questions of the group.

Until that day in 1987, I had always led wonderful study sessions—and I had done so countless times. But that memorable moment during Lent, sitting around an adult Sunday school room in Atlanta, with the windows open and the fragrance of the blooming azaleas drifting into the room, I failed. The session was a dud. I don't remember what introductory tidbit I led with or even what text we discussed. I just remember that sinking feeling that nothing was going on, the conversation had stalled.

I couldn't even sense God in the room anymore. The men seemed to have turned in on themselves, incapable or at least refusing to open their minds and hearts to the scriptures, the spirit, and to me. I was crestfallen—and desperate to regain the room. I finally asked, "Why do you bother to come here?" I had meant the question to be about Bible study in general and, more specifically, my session.

But when one man finally looked at me, with genuine sadness in his eyes, he gave an answer to a much broader question. "I come to church because I want to belong," he said. "I am looking for something greater than myself—something bigger that I can belong to." That man, in his longing for intentional community, changed the conversation and transformed the discussion—if you can call the awkward stumbling prior to that point a discussion.

Whenever I think of intentional community, I think of this and other churches I have attended in my life. Each church has enlarged my sense of God, though sometimes that has been through my disagreement with what has been preached from the pulpit. I experience community as the interaction with others, hearing the music, singing the hymns, and praying together. Though I have attended mainly Methodist churches, twice in my life I participated in Episcopal communities. The ritual, the incense, the chanting lifted the entire community into the light, I thought.

Connections Bigger than Oneself

Belonging to a community—something bigger than oneself and more than merely an association of individuals who share an interest—is important to most of us. In Abraham Maslow's famous hierarchy of human needs, belonging and love rank next in importance after meeting our most basic physiological needs (food, water, etc.) and safety.

> The most fundamental four layers of the pyramid contain what Maslow called "deficiency needs" or "d-needs": esteem, friendship and love, security, and physical needs. If these "deficiency needs" are not met—except for the most fundamental (physiological) need—there may not be a physical indication, but the individual will feel anxious and tense.[1]

Without belonging and love, we feel deprived, we experience anxiety and distress, perhaps we become incapable of cognitive learning, aesthetic appreciation, or real self-actualization. Maslow's theory is debatable, as most theories are, but in my experience real belonging is a fundamental need of human beings. People often find community and belonging within their families; among their friends; in clubs, teams, and Facebook groups; and in religious groups. Deep down, I believe we seek community as a way of belonging to something greater than ourselves.

While I was teaching at Candler School of Theology at Emory, I found community among my colleagues. Worship, unsurprisingly, was central to our life together. We experienced all different kinds of worship with different music, rituals, and theological approaches in sermons. We sat, we stood, and occasionally we danced. Our community's ultimate purpose was to learn and teach. We read papers together, we critiqued each other's work, we held each other accountable for standards of behavior in our teaching, writing, and community life. The elders in the community were called The Young Turks, a name given to them when they were in their 30s, though they were by that time in their 60s. They were all white men who had hired a diverse group of younger scholars as their colleagues. They were proud of us, encouraging us in our work. Jim Waits, Candler's dean and clearly our chief pastor, cared deeply for each one of us and for the community as a whole. His humor, his care, and his leadership made us more than simply an association of people doing similar things.

A Cultivator of Community

While teaching at Candler, I became a cultivator of community. I realized students learned best when I created intentional community in the classroom. Like the Bible studies I led, I made time for students to get to know each other and to know me. I created an environment where students could take risks and be imaginative. I delighted in helping these students grow in all sorts of ways, their minds and worlds enriched.

When I took my first administrative role as associate dean of Candler, I pledged myself to build community wherever I could. Later, at Colgate, then Swarthmore, I would find an already profound sense of community at these small liberal arts schools. So I focused on expanding diversity, with a focus on helping everyone find a sense of belonging. Every liberal arts college has its own rituals, and I wanted to make sure these rituals contributed to shared goals of learning and flourishing for all members of the community.

When I arrived at DU, I launched a listening tour. I had done this elsewhere and found it to be a great opportunity to hear what people liked about the place, what they wanted to see changed, and what they would never want to change. I would talk with students, staff, faculty, alumni, parents, and local leaders—anyone and everyone who contributed to the institution's community. DU is a teaching and research university of about 12,000 students, half graduate students and half undergraduates. Staff and faculty live all around the Denver metro area.

An almost-universal consensus emerged in the listening tour: everyone craved a stronger sense of community, more connection across the university, and a greater sense of institutional identity. Everyone wanted to learn more and belong more.

Building community became a theme throughout my time at DU. We created a "One DU" campaign to meet this need. It led to new rituals, like a new alumni event to celebrate and recognize our graduates. We put out Adirondack chairs across campus to encourage people to gather on the beautiful lawns. We brought in food trucks and hosted pop-up parties. We replaced a dark and uninviting student center with a stunning new Community Commons building that had a rooftop garden and gathering area that faced the mountains. We rethought how students lived together on campus and how they used their time to cultivate a stronger community. All of this contributed to higher rates of student success.

My Greatest Pride

I love building community. It is part of what makes me *Rebecca*. Of all the accomplishments in my life, I take greatest pride in the times I helped build communities. Sometimes the projects I completed seem small, like organizing sack lunches at Swarthmore where staff could hear faculty members speak. But those lunches created bonds between faculty and staff, allowed staff to get to know one another in new ways, and allowed them to benefit from the richness of the faculty knowledge. Other times, the projects were much bigger, like the building of the Inn at Swarthmore, where coworkers now gather after work and townspeople come to eat and drink.

Feeling the Loss

Despite the fact that the community makes me *me*, I am at a loss for it now. It is perhaps the one area where I have not found a completely fulfilling path forward.

I lost the profound sense of college and university community when I retired. I want a new church community, but haven't found one since our most recent move. I live in an area that contains some relatively large nondenominational communities. I suppose they have their own sense of ritual, but I miss the one I came to know in the smaller churches I served at various times. And while loud music with drums and electric guitars help many connect better to God, it makes it hard for me to quiet my heart and find peace. In the Rocky Mountain west, few churches have stained glass, and I never realized how much that meant to me until I moved here.

Some of my neighbors who have attended their church for 30 years say their long-term church friendships have endured no matter whether the weekly services they attend are online or in person. Other neighbors downplay the relationship aspect of attending a church; they go because they believe they are supposed to. But I long for a face-to-face community that worships, learns, feasts, and serves together.

The loss and longing of the community makes me sad. I really do feel like I have lost an essential part of myself. I worry I am too picky, too stuck in my ways, or even too lazy. I wonder if the ease and prevalence of Zoom in a post-COVID world has made it harder to find the type of face-to-face community I seek.

I imagine Christian communities, as well as other types, are being shaped in new ways that I haven't seen or experienced yet. I hope I will discover new forms of connection before my sense of self disappears.

How Can You Create a Sense of Belonging?

For me, making connections to something larger than myself came through my work bringing people together on college and university campuses and by participating in church communities. Admittedly, I haven't yet found the answers for myself on how to develop and maintain a sense of belonging now that my previous pathways are no longer open to me. But I haven't given up, and I hope you won't either. For as long as you can, continue to connect with people and with issues larger than yourself. It's a fundamental human need.

18

Tending the Garden of My Friends

"Now friendship possesses many splendid advantages,
but of course the finest thing of all about it is that it sends
a ray of hope into the future, and keeps our hearts from
faltering or failing by the wayside."[1]

—CICERO

BOTH MY GRANDMOTHERS LOVED their gardens. Grandma Gertie lived on a farm while I was growing up and had an enormous vegetable garden. She loved her cucumbers, carrots, potatoes, peas, beans, and everything else she could grow in that fertile soil. As a girl, I helped her weed the garden during the summers when I visited her and my grandpa Frank on their farm in tiny Narka, Kansas. I remember the relentless morning sun as we weeded. And, after dinner was done and the dishes were put away, we would be back in the garden, again fighting those weeds. Rows upon rows of vegetables, constantly under attack from a seemingly endless army of weeds. I always admired how much she loved that growing space. When the vegetables were ready to be harvested, she would receive the bounty. And all year long, I loved the pickles and sauerkraut, homemade from her own garden.

Grandma Theresa (Mac), meanwhile, lived in the same town as we did. She was a master gardener, and her backyard overflowed with flowers. Every time I visited her, until she went into the nursing home with Alzheimer's, I spent hours in the backyard with her. She also grew African violets in her basement and roses all around her house. I loved those flowers. The variety of colors, petals, smells, and stalks fascinated me. I would beg her to tell me about each one.

The roses were luscious to smell but prickly. The daylilies were bright and proud but lasted for only a brief time each year. The marigolds were protective of all the other flowers, short but mighty. The morning glories were tall, delicate, full of colors—great to make dolls to play with. And the lilacs: I could just fall into them, and they would always surround me with their love. Roses were (and still are) my favorite. They come in so many colors and have delightful names. I know they are prickly, but it makes them interesting and reminds me to be respectful. My grandmother won prizes for her roses because they were so special.

Over time, I came to imagine each flower to be like a friend. And now I find that the situation is reversed: I've come to see each of my friends as a unique flower in my friendship garden.

The Flowers in My Friendship Garden

I have always loved having friends. Since I was a small child, friends have delighted me. I find them fun, enjoyable, lovely, and each one a special prize in my life. My heart grieves when I think of forgetting my friends—losing the memories of our shared experiences and all that I learned from each one.

As a girl, my best friend was Marta Manning. We could play for hours and hours with our dolls. Sometimes one of our mothers would drape a bedsheet or quilt over the table and we would spend all afternoon playing in our "house." Marta saw things in our dolls that I didn't and vice versa. We could create adventures together, and it really took both of us to develop these adventures.

My family loves to point out that most of my friends are a bit eccentric, just like the prickly and beautiful roses I love so much. I had one dear friend at Colgate, Paul Schupf, an art collector, who just could not get along with anyone! Paul, now deceased, and I would go out to dinner every other week or so. We got along famously, and I learned so much about art and higher education from him, as he had served on numerous boards of liberal arts colleges. To most people, he showed only his thorns; to me, he revealed a glimpse of his deep knowledge and genuine delight in art and education. Maybe he was the most eccentric of my friends in his collection of art, his choice to be a financial investor based in Hamilton, New York (the town where Colgate University is located), instead of New York City, and his absolutely odd taste in nearly everything except fine wine. But I agree with my family: most of my friends are a bit more eccentric than most.

I am like a mermaid in that I prefer depth over shallowness when it comes to my friendships. All the years I worked, I learned to enjoy small talk. But left to my own, I much prefer to talk about what people love, what they would die for, who they think God is. Tom Frank writes poetry that I love to hear and shares his deep knowledge of church architecture. Barbara Brooks is an adventuress, and I learn so much from the way she pushes her comfort zone. Rosanna is my dance partner and *compañero* in justice.

A Portrait Gallery of Friends

When I first learned to paint portraits, I had a magnificent dream that I would paint as many of my dearest friends as I could and write what I have learned from them as a short tribute to each. As my mind grew fuzzy, I imagined, I would surround myself with the portraits, and my caretakers could read what I had learned from them or what I loved most about them. When I passed away, my friends could have the portraits, I thought. The first time I tried, I failed. The second time, I failed again. I admire people who can paint pictures of those they love; I intend to keep trying.

Susan Shapiro and I met in 1977 when we were both in graduate school at Chicago. Susan and I have talked at least once a week, and often more, since then. She is brilliant about religion, a wonderful teacher, and the single best listener I know. Her giggle makes me laugh. For years, my son called her "Aunt Susan."

John Witte and Eliza Ellison are the only real couple friends that Fred and I have. Our lives are so intertwined that we are more family than friends. Eliza's deep wisdom and wit and John's incredible knowledge of law and religion, as well as his amazing steadfastness as a friend, have taught both of us so much about life and love.

Serene Jones has a sheer intellectual courage and personal guts that have allowed her to accomplish so much. We see each other rarely and never talk in between, and yet we fall into each other's arms easily like I once fell into those lilacs of my grandmother's.

Ed Rowe has been a co-conspirator of mine in so many things. Years in age separate us, yet we have been so bonded since we met. Ed is a great writer and has always improved my writing. He was the first collaborator I worked with on this book. He was very patient drawing out my stories and helping to get words down on the page; I hope to learn some of his patience.

Gail O'Day, whom I tried to paint and failed, passed away too young. She and I taught together and hosted more dinner parties than I can count. I knew I could trust Gail to tell me the truth—always. I learned a lot about John, the Gospel, from her. She showed me what it means to be friends and, in particular, to be friends with God.

Murray Decock sends me his compositions and his bagpipe videos; he is a man who does well at whatever he tries to do, including being a deeply caring and honest friend.

Frances Lucas, Susan Henry-Crowe, Alicia Franck, and I still rock and roll more than 35 years after breaking the glass ceiling at Emory University. Thanks to them for pushing me to break yet another barrier.

My Grace Sisters, who I Marco Polo with all the time, have laughed with me, cried with me, thought with me, and shared their love with me. We live across the country, are different ages, and run in very different circles, and yet we are all deep friends.

I'm also blessed that new friends delightfully continue to appear in my life. Barbara Kreisman (the second Barbara mentioned in this book) retired on the same day as I did. When we were both working, we would find ourselves at the same receptions and would connect in marvelous ways. But only when we retired could we become friends. Barbara started a book club called The Untamed Women, and invited me into a bigger circle of friends who discuss challenging and fun books. We also share our challenges and our practices of joy. My new neighborhood has brought new friends: Pam Kaweske, Joyce Hall, Ruth Edmundson, and others. For the first time in my life I feel like I belong to something akin to a sorority. Women over 70 can still form such a thing!

And so it goes. So many wonderful friends in my garden to love, cherish, nurture and be nurtured by, and to respect and from whom to learn.

Weeding the Garden

My neurologist warned me that I should stay away from stress and try to limit the energy I spend in social engagement, but at the same time "make sure you keep your social connections." That was the challenge: limit social engagements but keep social connections!

I knew that I would need to make some adjustments. Although going to large events attended by dozens or hundreds of strangers made my head buzz from sensory overload, I could still delight in connecting with people I knew. I decided on keeping friendships when I could and maybe even making new ones.

But I also knew the advice meant that I had to weed my garden of friends a bit, avoiding people who are taxing and can only talk of themselves. A few friends had become somewhat toxic, always critical of me or way too negative about the world. Some friendships have lost their depth, and I can no longer stand just chatting about the weather or, worse yet, what someone had for dinner last night.

Weeding has been a slow process and hard, as I still love these friends, but I had to do it for my health. I need fewer friends now than I did at other times in my life. I am grateful to keep the ones with whom I thrive.

Blessed in My Friendships

Even after my weeding efforts, someone recently said to me, "You have lots of friends." It's true. I am a blessed woman. My friends, old and new, are my greatest teachers as well as companions of my heart. Friends are both a social and intellectual connection for me, keeping my soul and brain ever expanding and ever challenged. This ever-changing garden of friends with whom I have deep and abiding connection are another thing that makes me *me*.

What Gardens Will You Tend?

It seems that everything I recommend in this book should be accompanied by the caution "within your own capabilities and limitations." That is as true here of social connections as for anything else I've written about. Maintaining a garden of friendship is how I've chosen to expend my (limited) energy to achieve the goal of creating social connections. What gardens can you tend that will do the same for you? Perhaps that will be growing closer to family, or, like me, reaching out to friends for comfort and joy.

PART VI

What Next?

AT SOME POINT, I MAY FORGET that I have Alzheimer's, but the disease won't forget me. I cannot ignore the reality of Alzheimer's. I now sleep 12 hours a day. Sleep is wonderful, but despite my new-found appreciation for sleeping, I haven't fully shaken the feeling that I am squandering a lot of time: there is no escaping that my days are shorter now. And even when I wake up after 12 hours, it takes me another hour to get going. I can drive around where I live, but I can't drive into the city anymore. How long will I be able to drive at all? I can read and understand a book, but I often forget it within a week or so. I used to be able to recite paragraphs from obscure German philosophers I had read 20 years before. Those holes in my brain are taking up more space, and memories are escaping into them. They are my own special black holes.

My short-term forgetfulness can be funny, sometimes leading me to go up and down the stairs three times before I remember what I am looking for. But the memory loss can also be hard. I've put ice cream (that my family eats, not me!) in the pantry and the salad I made for dinner in the freezer.

I still hate thinking about not being able to feed myself, not getting to choose my clothes or being able to button them. With grim humor,

I try to console myself that at some point I will just eat all the ice cream I want. Something to look forward to, at least.

Every day I face the haunting questions: How soon and how quickly will the disease progress? For how much longer will I still be Rebecca?

The answer to both questions is that nobody knows.

So I face the questions that confront every person with Alzheimer's: *What next? How can I move forward?*

In the next chapters, I'll recap some lessons that are giving me the confidence to carve a path into the future knowing I'm doing everything I can to live fully as myself for as long as I can. Then I'll offer some simple advice for anyone else who has been diagnosed with the disease.

19

The Latest
(and Last?) Reinvention
of Rebecca Chopp

IN DECEMBER 2021, *The Chronicle of Higher Education* ran an article entitled "The Reinvention of Rebecca Chopp." Journalist Megan Zahneis captured the essentials of my life story with clarity and brilliance. The article demonstrated what an Alzheimer's diagnosis meant for someone who not only understood herself as a brain with a body attached, but also had spent so much of her career leading some of the nation's most prestigious colleges and universities. Zahneis ended the article with this sentence: "She's reinvented herself so many times. This, she knows, is one more reinvention."

I can't say this latest and perhaps last reinvention is more radical than becoming a minister after being raised in a non-churched home, or a professor and then administrator after being raised by parents who wouldn't support my going to college. Though the ending of this reinvention will be tragic, I can't say it has been more challenging than moving from the University of Chicago in Hyde Park to the culturally different world of Atlanta when I took an appointment at Emory University.

Each reinvention has enriched me. I have discovered new sides of my personality, grown in new ways, and enlarged my worldview. Moving to upstate New York to be president of Colgate brought out my inner party girl and athlete, which had been hidden even to me. Moving to Denver confirmed my deep-seated but neglected belief that I am a bit of a cowgirl at heart. This perhaps final reinvention has allowed me to see the world differently: through painting and an appreciation for details of color, light, and shadow; through developing new dimensions of my spirituality, including creating contemplative practices. Through finding new gifts such as the practice of mindfulness in diet; expanding my exercises; bonding with my dog; and, yes, sleeping more than I ever have before. I have reinvented myself as an Alzheimer's advocate and, in writing this nonacademic book, I have revealed more of myself than ever before.

This ability to continue to reinvent myself—to learn about and adapt to changes in my life—heartens me. It makes me feel less like I am destined to drift quickly into oblivion.

I still dread my Hades—the particular kind of death sentence where I will lose my mind, my memories, and myself, likely all before my body begins to fail. I remain scared of getting lost, gazing out the window for hours, being led around by others.

But—importantly—I was not (and am not) in Hades yet. I'm still alive, still reinventing, still learning new ways to live the most rewarding life I can. I'm still fighting as hard as I can to not just maintain the real me but continue to grow.

In this chapter, I wanted to summarize some of the important lessons that are helping me with this latest reinvention in hope they will inspire you to do the same.

1. Facing the Diagnosis with Gumption

Dealing with Alzheimer's is not for the faint hearted. It takes gumption—a mixture of common sense and initiative—to live as full a life as you can for as long as you can.

The lack of information about Alzheimer's disease, the stigma surrounding it, and the lack of information about how to live with it are the chains that keep us in darkness and shadows.

Obtaining a diagnosis is not an easy path—the science is still unclear, and I documented the struggles I went through trying to find a doctor who could give me straight answers. And life doesn't necessarily get easier with a diagnosis, either. The darkness that descends upon receiving the news is unmistakable and unavoidable. A few caregivers have told me they felt relieved to know the diagnosis, as it gave a name to what was happening with their loved ones. I understand and respect that reaction. But I didn't even have that brief response of relief, nor did Fred.

One challenge, though, is that during the process of discovery, the world around you keeps moving. For me, it felt like living in two worlds. I had to keep showing up to work, pretending all was normal, while repressing the knowledge and emotions around the diagnosis process.

But in hindsight, I'm grateful for the angst of an early diagnosis because it meant I learned about the disease that is affecting me while I was still aware and active enough to do something about it. Fred and I had to plan for a future that neither of us could even begin to comprehend, let alone come to terms with, but because of my early diagnosis, I could fully participate in making important and life-altering decisions. Fred and I made sure our legal documents were in place. We examined our finances and even moved not once, but twice trying to find the right fit in terms of where we could live most comfortably given our circumstances. All these decisions had to be made while

I was in shock and despair. But at least I was fully able to participate in the decision-making process.

While it was hard to retire much earlier than I had planned to do so, freeing myself from the stress of being a university chancellor allowed me to slow progress of the disease. I recognize not everyone can afford to retire early. But stress can be minimized, both through lifestyle changes and by employers' willingness to modify jobs and make reasonable accommodations for those with an Alzheimer's diagnosis.

I've always believed that knowledge is power. Now, I've learned that it takes courage to seek out that knowledge and wield the power.

2. Using Creativity and Spirituality to Push past the Darkness

I think I've been clear that getting a diagnosis of Alzheimer's leads to heaps of despair, depression, and fear. I want to be clear about this for two reasons. First, I don't want anyone thinking I am a Pollyanna who believes that Alzheimer's patients can *simply* live with joy. It takes a lot of work to get to that point. Second, by being forthright about my own struggles, I want to encourage others to talk about theirs in real time as the challenges appear.

I realize now I did not do as much as I could have in terms of being open about my diagnosis with others. It's not like losing a loved one, where well-wishers drop by your house to check on how you're doing. With an Alzheimer's diagnosis, no one knows what to say, so many people retreat. It seemed as though almost everyone who knew I had Alzheimer's assumed that I would spiral downward quickly—and they didn't know how to deal with it.

As you've read in this book, however, I am fighting still to push past this darkness and live in the light as much as possible. The more I practice simply being open to awe and grace, the more light I experience.

I still lament, but now it is often with others crying and occasionally cursing this dreadful disease. The beast of darkness and fear rears its head at night, so I tell myself stories of courageous heroes and sheroes before I sleep. And I have several pictures of saints hanging by my bed. Your spiritual way will no doubt be different.

Creativity has been another outlet that brings light into life. It has given me meaning and provided a depth I am not sure I have ever felt before, at least not in this way. And please take note that I didn't get to this point on my own. I was lucky to have a messenger from the gods, by the name of Frances, who flew in and insisted I had to learn to paint. Despite my resistance, I did learn to paint. And it didn't take me long to find myself having fun, lost for hours at a time in the process of painting. Painting stretched my mind, and it brought joy. Who could have imagined that I'd ever find *fun* again? Certainly not me—not at first.

Creativity in any form is good for us, good for our brains, our souls, our world. Creativity stretches your brain, fuels the soul, and brings peace. There is still time to rediscover your creative self if, like so many of us, you have lost it in adulthood. Maybe you will sing or learn crafts. Maybe you will restore cars or learn to knit. Or learn to garden: I envy gardeners and how patient they must be to plant the bulbs and wait for the brilliant burst of colors they had imagined from the beginning. Find something creative you like to do, and just do it!

This is a time to be open to the nonrational (spirituality) and the nonlinear (creativity). Approach this with curiosity, and enjoy what you experience.

3. Treating My Body Well

I am eternally grateful to Dr. Hudson, who as my neurologist inspired me to believe there was some hope. And to Dr. Granholm-Bentley—Lotta—my friend who studies Alzheimer's and became the bridge to get me out of Hades. They sent me on the most important research project of my life: finding out all I could about Alzheimer's disease and about how to mitigate its hideous effects through lifestyle changes that range from creativity to spirituality to taking care of my body. I have learned that the brain–body connection is powerful. Even as Alzheimer's erodes the function of the brain, some of the best ways to hang on to consciousness—to meaningful and joyful living—as long as possible is to treat your entire body well.

So to keep living in the light, I have to stay healthy. And to stay healthy, I have to follow my doctor's orders. I think there is no doubt that physical well-being can help hold off the darkness.

Since I am not very good with orders, which run counter to my rebellious spirit, I had to use the story of Pericles to help me reframe my doctor's orders as gifts. (I don't know how you will reframe orders if you resist orders as I have always done, but if you find something that works for you, I would love to know!)

Pericles had an unbreakable sword to kill off the mad Medusa. Though my demons cannot be so easily vanquished, I can work hard at holding them off as with Athena's shield. Winged sandals help me fly through exercise, diet, and sleep.

I exercise a lot; it is a luxury of retirement. I live in a beautiful location near the mountains, so walking and hiking are easy for me. But I also like to walk in urban areas where there is great people watching. Buhdy, my beloved dog, and I set no limits to where we will walk and hike. Though not intensive exercise, even this kind of moderate exercise is good for the brain and body. Some researchers still swear that 10,000 steps a day is the key to long-term health.

I tend to be most impressed with the research that promotes intensive cardio to the point where it is hard to talk while biking or walking uphill. I also trust the research that shows some type of resistance training or weightlifting is important. I really enjoy weightlifting. Several years ago, I could deadlift my husband's weight of 165 pounds. I weigh only 118 pounds! Now I am using moderately heavy weights for my size, but even very light weights and multiple repetitions count. Balance, flexibility, and coordination are important for Alzheimer's patients—and for everyone, especially as we age. I just started a Barre class at the gym in my over-55 community. All of us white- and gray-haired ladies are amazingly flexible thanks to this class.

The key is to find what you like: horseshoes, pickleball, mall walking, gardening, bike riding, kickboxing (Ruth Bader Ginsburg was taking kickboxing lessons in her 80s), golf, whatever gets you moving. Get your body moving so your brain can get stronger.

Diet is also critical. More and more research shows the good effects of a healthy diet, most especially the MIND diet. I am always amazed at how adaptive human beings are to different diets. Food is so different around the world, and yet we can move anywhere, and over time, we can adapt. In different historical periods our own ancestors ate quite differently than we do now. Food is fuel and pleasure. I love homemade frozen Greek yogurt with berries and walnuts. A really good chicken-veggie curry is great too. I have become a salmon salad lover. The trick is finding the foods that are on the MIND diet that you enjoy (or can learn to enjoy).

After lots of exercise, good food, doing something creative, and being attuned and open to ultimacy, you should be tired. I sure am! Sleep is such a blessing, and it is essential for clearing out those brain-killing toxins. I can sleep 12 hours at a time now—something I never imagined myself doing. Most of my life, I would have felt guilty since I wasn't working, cleaning the house, or whatever else one "should" be doing. Now educated about the importance of sleep and, of course, being retired, I sleep and I feel good about it. Sleep is a gift. Sleep is one order

I don't mind following. My doctor prescribed a low-dose sleeping pill, and I am happy to take it. The most important thing for you, and for me, is to sleep.

4. Holding On Tight to What Makes Me Me

In Part V, I talked about what makes me feel most like myself even as parts of me slip away. I am holding on to these aspects of my life as tightly as I can.

A lifetime of being interested in ethics and justice has led me to advocacy. I have become an Alzheimer's advocate. I write, I speak, I protest, I rally in support of Alzheimer's research and better treatment of Alzheimer's patients. I paint for the Alzheimer's Association Annual Purple Gala. I give interviews, do webinars, and talk to any group that will have me. I am still me and will advocate for as long as I can.

I see this work as an extension of my love of teaching, which, for me, is an act of love—love of knowledge, of empowerment, of participating in discovery, and of building community.

But I also think if I did nothing more than keeping open to the ultimate—God—as much as possible, I would be bringing good energy into the world. Maybe God needs more of us just spending time opening ourselves and, through ourselves, opening the world to grace.

Researchers and neurologists tell us social connections are important for our brains. Other people make us mentally and emotionally stretch, and the human-to-human connection seems to nurture us. Alzheimer's can be isolating. I worry about repeating myself, or in my case, lisping too much.

But for now, I am still me as I work to maintain friendships. Friends have been a part of my life forever. Some friendships fade. I have had to exit from some, and I continue to find new ones. Friends are people I trust, with whom I laugh, and to whom I can discuss anything. I also know I have a few friends who, like my family, will interact with me and tell me stories and share memories, even when I can no longer understand them.

Community has been another form of social connection that has and continues to be important for me. I don't know if it has to be important for everyone, especially if they have friends. But for me, belonging to a mission-oriented group has been a big part of my life for many years. As an educator, I worked hard to make the colleges and universities I served what I called intentional communities—centered around a clear mission, ultimately contributing to a better world.

The lives of my friends are as important to me as my own. I delight in hearing about grandchildren, travels, hobbies, and their dinners out with loved ones. I am eager to do all I can to support them in times of struggle and grief, or just those times where we have to sing the blues together. I can't imagine a reinvention of myself without having friends, and it saddens me to know that at some point my garden of friends will have to shrink even more than it has already.

As a minister and a theologian, I enjoy hearing the message of God, but it is not the most important part of belonging. To me, being a part of a religious community is about the people caring for one another, communing together, and living their lives in service to something greater than themselves. That is why what I have loved most has been belonging to a church, though that was not a part of my upbringing. I still enjoy boisterous potlucks and BBQs and coffee hours. I like Bible studies and book clubs where we discuss important things and not-so-important things. I like the services where we sing together, recite common liturgies, and attend to the presence of the ultimate together. But that is me. You, I hope, can find your own community.

Still Me, but Different

Taking care of the body, learning new ways of creativity, and expanding or developing spirituality is like reinventing yourself. I feel like a different me, and yet I am the same person.

The Alzheimer's path is different for everyone. I have met some people who always took care of their bodies but had to expand their creativity and develop their spirituality. Others have had the kind of faith that allows them to process this life-alternating news with grace and dignity . . . but they have had to learn to make exercise or a healthy diet a normal part of their lifestyle.

You have to find new stories to live with, and you have to reinvent your story. You have to be you, albeit perhaps a reinvented you.

I am Rebecca, and I have always liked to fight for justice (which I now apply to being an Alzheimer's advocate), have lots of friends (with a little weeding needed nowadays), and belong to communities. I have always enjoyed learning about Greek myths, not aware at the time that I would find in them the inspiration to shape the newest version of me. I like music and hiking, yet at the same time am finding new layers to my talents, interests, and abilities.

I don't know if I'm experiencing the final reinvention of Rebecca Chopp. In some ways, I hope not, because that would mean that I still have the wherewithal to continue to learn and adapt. Yet if another reinvention is part of my future, I know I will find myself returning to my core.

My friend Geri told me when I once interviewed her, "I want people to understand I am still me." I've encountered this same sentiment time and again reading books and articles by people with Alzheimer's. Even as our symptoms advance—no longer able to drive, unable to speak as well as before, maybe no longer able to read books or solve puzzles—we are still our own unique selves.

Continuing the Fight

As I write this, it's August 2023, a full four-and-a-half years after I got my official diagnosis of Alzheimer's. It is also years beyond the doom that was foretold by the only neurologist who is not named in this book—the one who predicted that by this time I wouldn't be able to feed myself or button my shirt. I count the fact that I can do both those things as victories, not to mention the fact that I'm writing this book, have learned how to paint, and feel closer to the ultimate than ever before in my life.

Obviously, the worst of my nightmares have not come true. At least not yet. And I'm going to continue to fight to make sure they don't come true anytime soon.

20

Living Forward

I KNOW IT MAY SEEM ODD TO CONCLUDE a memoir about Alzheimer's by talking about the future, but it is so important for us who live with this disease and for our caregivers to believe there is a future that includes us. We who live with the disease should not be defined or confined by our diagnosis. We still live forward. Alzheimer's will most likely someday overtake us, unless a cure or miraculous treatment occurs. (It would need to happen in the very near future to help me.) But until then, we refuse to surrender, and we enjoy life every second that we can.

I end this book with three thoughts about living forward.

Find a Way to Tell Your Story

We need stories of our refusal to surrender. We need to raise awareness. Until recently, this disease has been diagnosed in most people only in the middle to the later stages, as it was with my grandmothers and my mother. There are few stories written by those of us with Alzheimer's. The world needs our stories: people need to hear us say that we are still *us*, and we are still here. Many organizations such as Voices of Alzheimer's have websites to tell our stories. Contact the Alzheimer's

Association and ask if you can be a speaker or meet with one of the care groups. I have found many care partners are eager to meet with me. Or just tell people in your neighborhood and your family about your story. Our stories will inspire. They will help slay the stigmas.

Pay Love Forward

You may feel limited in what you have to offer the world. While that may be true, one thing I've found that all of us have to offer is love to our family and friends. I express this love not only through words but also in spending time with the people who mean the most to me.

I am blessed with two incredible primary caretakers: my husband, Fred, and my son, Nate. My love for them shows through the pages of this book. Fred has always been "my home," my anchor, my laugh partner, my companion. As I progress more and more in the disease, he picks up more and more of the responsibilities of daily living. He cleans, manages the books, washes the clothes, and does the shopping. I still manage to cook some meals for us, but I know my cooking is not what it used to be. I forget lots of things, and Fred's mantra to himself is "It is not her fault, she doesn't remember, I love her." Until I cannot do so any longer, I want to love him actively. I want to pay forward all the care he will give and the love he will continue to share with me.

Nate and his wife, Lisa, recently moved nearby so he can be actively engaged in my care. Every time I thank him for it, he says, "Mom, I want to spend time with you." He drives me nearly everywhere, which allows me to see friends in Denver (30 miles away), go to the Botanic Gardens, visit museums, and even take trips. Nate is an artist and paints with me. He is an avid moviegoer, and while our tastes are slightly different, he never says no when I want to go to a movie. Lisa accompanies us when she can, and I have the joy of being with both of them. Since Fred's health is not great, it is a comfort to both Fred and me to know we can count on Nate and Lisa. I want to pay forward to Nate and Lisa, to do fun things with them and to enjoy them while I can. I want them to be filled with fun memories.

Kathy, my sister, and Bob, her husband, live in Denver. Kathy and I have always "played together," and we continue to do so. Always the protective older sister, she often told me I worked too hard. I guess I should have listened! Now we play—art, music, hiking, trips, lunches out. I want to pay forward for all she has done my entire life to make my life better.

I don't know who you want or need to pay forward. Set your intention every day to pay love forward.

Live with Joy

Looking ahead, I want to live with joy, as my neurologist suggested. As you've read many times in this book, joy for me is painting, praying, being with loved ones, seeing the flowers bloom in the spring, and walking with Buhdy. Joy is reading a good book, having lunch with a friend, experiencing the ultimate (God) anywhere I can. The ultimate is everywhere, so joy is having the eyes and ears and senses to experience the beauty of life.

Joy, I have learned in this experience, is not the opposite of despair or fear; all of those emotions coexist. I can worry about the state of this country and the world, be saddened by the deaths of children, be furious at the hatred and evil I see. But I can still feel joy. Not every second, but it is my intention to be joyous, even as I fret about my life and about the world.

While writing this book, Nate and I traveled to Atlanta. I hadn't been on an airplane since my diagnosis in 2019. COVID stopped air travel, my husband was ill, and I just didn't get around to traveling again for several years. I had also been constantly traveling in my career, so I needed a break. I got an invitation to visit with some friends in Atlanta, and Nate wanted to see his father, so off we went. I was nervous about the airport, but it all worked well. We had a wonderful visit. I was tired, but every moment visiting friends was worth it. We got to the airport to fly home and went out to the terminal. I remembered I needed some headphones for a podcast I was doing the next week. We stopped at a display that had them. The woman working there told us the display was closing but asked what we were looking for, found what we wanted, and announced they would be perfect. I purchased them, and as we walked away she shouted out to us, "Don't let anyone steal your joy."

My final words to you: **"Don't let anyone steal your joy."**

The Light

MURRAY DECOCK, A FRIEND AND COMPOSER, has been an ongoing thought partner in writing this book. Based on the chapters and on our conversations, he wrote a song he called "The Light" for me. The song expresses my dreams, my fears, my loves. It says in lyrics and music "still me." You can listen to the song on YouTube: (https://www.youtube.com/watch?v=AT-zUIclQtE).

The Light

I'm writing these words down
My mind is racing ahead
To finish this story
And share it before I forget.

As I fill up these pages
I'll just leave a few clues.
And together we'll read every chapter slowly
So these words will bring me back to you.

I'm painting a picture with memories I've saved
through the years.
So I've mixed all my colors,
To make sure that they won't disappear.

All these portraits I've painted
Are like flowers I've grown from a seed.
And every stroke of my brush is like
The sun's warming touch helping me . . .

Walk out of this darkness
And step in to the light.

Where they never expect us
To remember all that we've seen with our eyes.

Now I know how this day ends,
With a little more black than white.
But I never learned how to live in the dark and so
I'll just be the light.

I dream that I'm dancing
To music I still recognize,
When it's sung by the voices
Of people I've known across my whole life.

Faces of kindness.
Faces I see with my heart, not my eyes.
I hope they can stay for a while,
Just so I know that it's safe and then I'll . . .

Walk out of the darkness
And step in to the light,
Where they never expect us
To remember all that we've seen with our eyes.

Now I know how the day ends

With a little more black than white.

I won't lie awake. I won't hide.
And when the days turn to smoke and float by,
I can just turn to the heart of my life.

To walk out of this darkness
And step in to the light.
Where they never expect us
To remember all that we've seen with our eyes.

Now I know how the day ends
With a little more black than white.
But I never learned how to live in the dark and
So I'll just be the light.

An Unconcluded Postscript

As I finish this book, five years have passed since that visit to the primary care physician that led to my Alzheimer's diagnosis. I'm happy to report that very recently my neurologist told me my symptoms had not progressed very much. In fact, my prognosis is better now than I ever thought it could be. Wow!

After my neurologist told me I might live for many more years in my present condition, I walked out of her office and the light was brighter. My imagination exploded: "I think I will remodel my living room with bold colors," "I am going to Scotland and other places," "Maybe I will write a children's book about adventures with my dog." I laughed out loud: I have time to love and to advocate and to continue expanding my life rather than let it shrink.

Through my research and networking, I have met many people who, like me, refuse to surrender to the darkness that an Alzheimer's diagnosis can bring. Recently, one person said to me, his voice filled with joy, "I like myself now, I am a better husband, father, and friend." I understood exactly what he meant because I feel the same way.

Everyone's journey is different. What will help one person may not help another. And no matter what we do, the disease will eventually progress. But I want you all to embrace the proof that early detection coupled with lifestyle changes and medical treatment can enable you to slow it down.

Our attitude is everything, my friends! We cannot know how life will unfold, so let's live in the light as much as we can. Whether as patient, as caregiver, as lover, or as friend, let's keep our curiosity. Let's awaken our imaginations to possibilities instead of nightmares. I'm living proof that doing so can lead to an enriching life despite an Alzheimer's diagnosis.

Notes

Introduction

1. "Orphan Trains" were operated between 1854 and 1929 to relocate children who were orphans or whose parents could not support them. Children from eastern cities were placed on trains and relocated as far away as the Midwest and Texas. Children were expected to help around the house/farm and in return to be supported by the strangers with whom they were placed. Many, but certainly not all, of these children were treated as indentured servants. This system was a forerunner to today's system of foster care. "Orphan Train," Wikipedia, accessed September 12, 2023, https://en.wikipedia.org/wiki/Orphan_Train.

2. "CMS Announces Plan to Ensure Availability of New Alzheimer's Drugs," CMS.gov, June 1, 2023, https://www.cms.gov/newsroom/press-releases/cms-announces-plan-ensure-availability-new-alzheimers-drugs.

Chapter 5

1. Daniel Gibbs, *A Tattoo on My Brain: A Neurologist's Personal Battle against Alzheimer's Disease* (Cambridge, UK: Cambridge University Press, 2021).

2. Gibbs, *A Tattoo on My Brain*, 87.

Chapter 6

1. "Alzheimer's Disease," National Institutes of Health, accessed September 13, 2023, https://www.nih.gov/research-training/accelerating-medicines-partnership-amp/alzheimers-disease.

2. 2023 Alzheimer's Disease Facts and Figure, Alzheimer's Association, accessed September 13, 2023, https://www.alz.org/media/Documents/alzheimers-facts-and-figures.pdf.

3. "Alzheimer's Disease."

Chapter 7

1. The Art Sherpa (website), accessed September 14, 2023, https://theartsherpa.com.

Chapter 8

1. Betty Edwards, *Drawing on the Right Side of the Brain* (New York: TarcherPerigree, 2012), 35.

Chapter 10

1. Aretha Franklin, "Precious Lord," accessed September 14, 2023, https://www.youtube.com/watch?v=0Sl59Prs8CE.

Chapter 11

1. A recent *New York Times* article entitled "How a Bit of Awe Can Improve Your Health" by Hope Reese (Jan. 3, 2023) explains even more health benefits of awe, https://www.nytimes.com/2023/01/03/well/live/awe-wonder-dacher-keltner.html.

2. Anne Lamott, *Traveling Mercies: Some Thoughts on Faith* (New York: Anchor Books, 1999), 143.

Chapter 12

1. Johann Baptist Metz, *Faith in History and Society: Toward a Practical Fundamental Theology*, trans. David Smith (New York: Seabury Press, 1980), 207–208.

Part IV

1. Dean Sherzai, Alexander Sherzai, and Ayesha Sherzai, "Lifestyle Intervention and Alzheimer Disease," *Journal of Family Practice* 71, no. 1 (Supplement 1 Lifestyle, January/February 2022): eS83–eS89, doi: 10.12788/jfp.0286.

Chapter 13

1. Wendy Suzuki, "The Brain-Changing Benefits of Exercise," TEDWomen 2017, November 2017, https://www.ted.com/talks/wendy_suzuki_the_brain_changing_benefits_of_exercise/transcript.

2. See, for instance, Kirk I. Erickson, Michelle W. Voss, Ruchika Shaurya Prakash, Chandramallika Basak, Amanda Szabo, Laura Chaddock, Jennifer S. Kim et al., "Exercise Training Increases Size of Hippocampus and Improves Memory," *Proceedings of the National Academy of Sciences of the United States of America* 108, no. 7 (February 15, 2011): 3017–3022, doi: 10.1073/pnas.1015950108.

3. David H. Brown, *Beating the Dementia Monster: How I Stopped the Advance of Cognitive Impairment from Alzheimer's Disease* (CreateSpace, 2018), 75.

4. Suzuki, "The Brain-Changing Benefits of Exercise."

Chapter 14

1. The MIND acronym is short for a mouthful of syllables, "Mediterranean-DASH Intervention for Neurodegenerative Delay."

2. Dr. Martha Clare Morris, *Diet for the MIND: The Latest Science on What to Eat to Prevent Alzheimer's and Cognitive Decline* (New York: Little, Brown, 2017), 6–7.

3. Cheryl Mussatto, *The Nourished Brain: The Latest Science on Food's Power for Protecting the Brain from Alzheimers and Dementia* (Self-published, 2018), 37.

4. Maggie Moon, *The MIND Diet: A Scientific Approach to Enhancing Brain Function and Helping Prevent Alzheimer's and Dementia* (Berkeley, CA: Ulysses Press, 2016), 27.

Chapter 15

1. Rebecca Robbins, Stuart F. Quan, Matthew D. Weaver, Gregory Bormes, Laura K. Barger, and Charles A. Czeisler, "Examining Sleep Deficiency and Disturbance and Their Risk for Incident Dementia and All-Cause Mortality in Older Adults across 5 Years in the United States," *Aging* 13, no. 3 (February 11, 2021): 3254–3268, https://doi.org/10.18632/aging.202591.

2. A. Roger Ekirch, "Segmented Sleep in Preindustrial Societies," *Sleep* 39, no. 3 (March 1, 2016): 715–716, doi: 10.5665/sleep.5558.

3. "Why You Should Care About Free Radicals," Cleveland Clinic, July 19, 2022, https://health.clevelandclinic.org/free-radicals/.

4. Melonyce McAfee, "The Nap Bishop Is Spreading the Good Word: Rest," *The New York Times*, October 13, 2022, https://www.nytimes.com/2022/10/13/well/live/nap-ministry-bishop-tricia-hersey.html.

Part V

1. B. Smith and Dan Gasby with Michael Shnayerson, *Before I Forget: Love, Hope, Help, and Acceptance in Our Fight Against Alzheimer's* (New York: Penguin, 2016), 268.

Chapter 16

1. "Medusa: The Real Story of the Snake-Haired Gorgon, " Greek Mythology.com, accessed September 16, 2023, https://www.greekmythology.com/Myths/Creatures/Medusa/medusa.html.

Chapter 17

1. "Maslow's Hierarchy of Needs," Wikipedia, accessed September 16, 2023, https://en.wikipedia.org/wiki/Maslow%27s_hierarchy_of_needs.

Chapter 18

1. Cicero, "On Friendship," cited in Eudora Welty and Ronalds A Sharp, eds. *The Norton Book of Friendship* (New York: W.W. Norton, 1991), 71.

Acknowledgments

Thanks to my husband, Fred, and my son, Nate. Besides laughing with me and loving me, they take care of nearly everything. Nate convinced me in July 2022 that I had to write this book and write it in a way that could be read.

I want to thank my family and friends, whose loving support and challenging engagement continue to make life a fulfilling adventure. You know who you are and how deep your support of this book means to me.

The Morgridge Family Foundation supported the writing and publishing of this book. Without the generosity of their support, a generosity that gave me an incredible push, the book would have been extremely difficult to write, let alone publish. Barbara Brooks, director of publishing and communications, and friend of many years, advocated for the project and then held my hand at all points. She provided me with great editorial, professional, and personal support.

Ed Rowe, my co-conspirator of many years, generously agreed to edit this before it went to the press. He also pushed me to unpack my experiences, express my feelings, and paint pictures with words.

Richard Nodell, Murray Decock, Susan Shapiro, Ralph Patrick, and Rosanna Panizo brought their expertise and deep engagement in reading drafts, often helping me clarify my thoughts and always to push deeper.

Shanna Cullen is my fitness trainer and much more. She has taught me so much about the brain–body connection, motivation, and healthy nutrition. She has kept me strong.

Researchers of Alzheimer's disease, especially Lotta Granholm-Bentley, have been invaluable teachers and supporters. Along with the many doctors and other Alzheimer's specialists mentioned in this book, I have been blessed with good advice.

The Voices of Alzheimer's Team: Jim and Geri Taylor, Phil Gutis, Jay Reinstein, LuPita Gutierrez-Parker, and Terrie Montgomery have been my A Team in many ways, including my avenue for activism. To the additional members of the board: George Vradenburg, Meryl Comer, Sue Peschin, John Dwyer, and Pamela Price: thank you for providing me so many opportunities to test out ideas.

The Alzheimer's Association has provided me wonderful opportunities to learn and lead, and resources to keep learning. What an honor it is to work with such dedicated and knowledgeable individuals in this organization. Special thanks to Jim Herlihy and Ralph Patrick.

Finally, I want to thank my amazing team at Greenleaf. Everyone at this press has been effective, efficient, and supportive. Special thanks to Sue Reynard, my editor, who made this book more readable and more interactive (and sent me pictures of crop art!).

About the Author

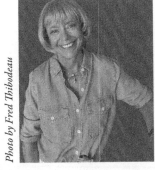

Photo by Fred Thibodeau

REBECCA S. CHOPP, PHD, is an Alzheimer's activist and educator. After retiring in 2019 due to an Alzheimer's diagnosis, Chopp co-founded Voices of Alzheimer's. Today, she serves as a member of the board of directors and the early-stage advisory board of the national Alzheimer's Association, and is a former member of the board of the Colorado Chapter of the Alzheimer's Association. Chopp is a frequent speaker and writer on timely diagnosis, research for a cure, access and affordability of drugs, and lifestyle intervention for those with Alzheimer's.

Before Chopp's diagnosis, she was a widely published author and editor, an ordained minister, and a renowned academic in the fields of education, philosophy, religion, and feminism. Chopp served as the 18th, and first female, chancellor of the University of Denver. She has served in leadership positions at Swarthmore College, Colgate University, Emory University, and Yale University. Since retiring, Chopp devotes every day to living with joy. She enjoys painting classical portraits and abstracts, hiking with her dog, reading, and spending time with family and friends.